Heada

More than 40 million Americans suffer from chronic headaches. Pharmaceutical drugs might temporarily subdue the
pain, but they can be habit-forming and come with worri-
some side effects. Moreover, the headaches keep coming
back.

Master herbalist David Hoffmann will help you target
the underlying cause of your headaches—whether stress-
or hormone-induced, a result of food allergy or a by-
product of a sinus infection. Then he suggests the appropriate herbal remedies or lifestyle solutions to heal and
balance the body so that headache pain can soften and
disappear once and for all.

About the Author

As a member of Britain's National Institute of Medical Herbalists, David Hoffmann has been a phytotherapist for almost 20 years. He is Assistant Professor of Integral Health Studies at the California Institute of Integral Studies, is a founding member and past president of the American Herbalist Guild and was director of the California School of Herbal Studies. The author of nine books on herbalism, his second book, *The New Holistic Herbal*, has become a standard text and has been translated into eight languages. Mr. Hoffmann teaches phytotherapy at schools throughout the English-speaking world. He is the author also of *Herbs to Relieve Stress*, another Keats Good Herb Guide.

A KEATS GOOD HERB GUIDE

HERBS TO RELIEVE HEADACHES

David Hoffmann

Keats Publishing, Inc.   New Canaan, Connecticut

HERBS TO RELIEVE HEADACHES

Copyright © 1997 by David Hoffmann

All Rights Reserved

No part of this book may be reproduced in any form without the written consent of the publisher.

Library of Congress Cataloging-in-Publication Data

Hoffmann, David, 1951–
    Herbs to relieve headaches / David Hoffmann.
        p.   cm.—(A Keats Good Herb Guide)
    Includes bibliographical references and index.
    ISBN 0-87983-766-7
    1. Headache—Alternative treatment. 2. Herbs—Therapeutic use.
I. Title.   II. Series.
    RB128.H64   1996
    616.8'49106—dc21   96-47003
                                                                    CIP

Printed in the United States of America

Good Herb Guides are published by
Keats Publishing, Inc.
27 Pine Street (Box 876)
New Canaan, Connecticut 06840-0876

98 97 96   6 5 4 3 2 1

Contents

What Are Headaches and What Causes Them?

Headaches, one of the most common health problems affecting humanity, are among the 10 most common symptoms for which medical advice is sought, accounting for 18 million outpatient visits a year in the United States.[1] More than 40 million Americans suffer from chronic headaches without regard to race, culture, lifestyle, occupation or geography. For at least half of these people, the problem is severe and sometimes disabling. In addition to loss of productivity, billions of dollars are spent on various forms of treatment and habituation to medications, plus the resulting family and work problems are significant. Despite their prevalence, headaches aren't simply the by-product of a modern, fast-paced society. Medical records left by ancient cultures from the Orient to the New World describe headaches.

WHY DOES IT HURT?

What hurts in a headache? Several areas of the head can hurt, including those affected by a network of nerves extending over the scalp and by certain nerves in the face, mouth and throat. Also sensitive to pain, because they contain delicate nerve fibers, are the muscles of the head and blood vessels found along the surface and at the base of the brain. The bones of the skull and tissues of the brain itself, however, never hurt because they lack pain-sensitive nerve fibers.

Pain is a complex experience consisting of a physiological response to a "painful" stimulus followed by an emotional response. It is a warning mechanism that helps to protect us and is primarily associated with injury, or the threat of injury, to bodily tissues. But headache pain is different. For most headaches, even when the pain is severe, there is no underlying disease—not even a brain tumor.

The point at which a stimulus begins to become painful is the pain perception threshold; most studies have found this point to be relatively similar among disparate groups. However, the pain tolerance threshold, the point at which pain becomes unbearable, varies significantly. Childhood experiences, cultural attitudes, genetic makeup and gender are factors that contribute to the development of each individual's perception of and response to different types of pain. Although some people may be able to physiologically withstand pain better than others, cultural factors rather than heredity usually account for this ability.

Your head can ache in a variety of ways:

- **Severity.** The pain can range from mild to excruciating, annoying to incapacitating.
- **Frequency and duration.** It can strike occasionally or daily, lasting a few minutes to hours or days.
- **Related symptoms.** It can be accompanied by other problems, such as nausea or vomiting.
- **Location.** The pain can be localized in one spot or it can affect the entire head.

When to Have Your Headaches Evaluated

About 90 percent of all headaches are *not* caused by a serious disorder and can be treated effectively with herbal pain relievers alone or in combination with rest, ice packs or a variety of relaxation techniques. However, there are certain symptoms that should be regarded as indicators that a competent medical diagnosis is called for. These include:

- Sudden, severe headache.
- Headache associated with convulsions.
- Headache accompanied by confusion or loss of consciousness.
- Headache following a blow to the head.
- Headache associated with pain in the eye or ear.
- Persistent headache in a person who was previously headache-free.
- Recurring headache in children.
- Headache that interferes with normal life.
- Headache that occurs three or more times per week.
- Headache that worsens over a period of weeks or months.
- Headache following a head or neck injury.
- Headache that begins after age 50.
- Headache accompanied by blurred vision or slurred

speech, numbness, weakness or loss of feeling in a limb.

- Headache accompanied by confusion or drowsiness.
- Headache accompanied by fever, nausea, shortness of breath or vomiting, and/or unexpected symptoms that affect the eyes, ears, nose or throat.
- Headache that is precipitated by exertion such as exercise, coughing, sneezing or bending over.

The Varieties of Headaches

Headaches brought on by muscle spasms are classified as tension headaches; those caused by the dilation of blood vessels are called vascular headaches. A more specialized classification by the International Headache Society further divides headaches into 14 categories. A system that helps the herbalist select the appropriate remedy divides headaches into these groupings:

- **Environmental.** Caused by pollutants, body posture, lighting, sound, etc.
- **Stress.** Physical, emotional or mental upset.
- **Dietary.** Possible allergy to certain foods, medications or additives e.g. xanthine-containing foods.
- **Organic.** Caused by a disease such as hypertension.

Pain may also be referred to the head (i.e., felt in the head even though the site of disease is elsewhere) by eye disorders such as glaucoma and refractive errors, infections or tumors of the nasal sinuses, dental infections and arthritis of the neck.

MUSCLE CONTRACTION AND TENSION HEADACHES

These are continuous and generalized pains felt from front to back or all around the head and are generally less severe than migraines. The pain is usually a dull ache that has been described as feeling like a tight band around the head. A tension headache can be simply a feeling of pressure or severe enough to cause painful knots in neck and scalp muscles. While emotional stress and letdown after such stress are the most common causes, arthritis of the joints of the neck may also contribute. Tension headaches alone are also often experienced by migraine sufferers, and a combined form of headache can also occur.

Tension headache is named not only for the role of stress in triggering the pain, but also for the contraction of neck, face and scalp muscles brought on by stressful events. Tension headache is a severe but temporary form of muscle contraction headache. The headache usually disappears after the period of stress is over.

By contrast, chronic muscle contraction headaches can last for weeks, months and sometimes years. The pain of these headaches is often described as a tight band around the head or a feeling that the head and neck are in a cast. The pain is steady and is usually felt on both sides of the head. Chronic muscle contraction headaches can cause sore scalps; even combing one's hair can be painful.

Occasionally, muscle contraction headaches are accompanied by nausea, vomiting and blurred vision, but there is no preheadache syndrome as with migraine. Muscle contraction headaches have not been linked to hormones or foods, as has migraine, nor is there a strong hereditary connection.

For many people, chronic muscle contraction headaches are caused by depression and anxiety. These people tend to get their headaches in the early morning or evening when conflicts in the office or home are anticipated. Depression and anxiety have also been noted to lower both the pain perception and pain tolerance thresholds; anger or excitement, however, can obscure or lessen pain temporarily.

Emotional factors are not the only triggers of muscle-contraction headaches. Certain physical postures—such as holding one's chin down while reading—can lead to head and neck pain. Tensing head and neck muscles during sexual excitement can also cause headache. So can prolonged writing under poor light, holding a phone between the shoulder and ear, or even gum chewing.

More serious problems that can cause muscle contraction headaches include degenerative arthritis of the neck and temporomandibular joint dysfunction or TMJ. TMJ is a disorder of the joint between the temporal bone (above the ear) and the mandible or lower jaw bone. The disorder results from poor bite and jaw clenching.

Treatment for muscle contraction headache varies. The first consideration is to treat any specific disorder or disease that may be causing the headache. For example, arthritis of the neck is treated with anti-inflammatory herbs, and TMJ may be helped by corrective devices for the mouth and jaw. People who suffer infrequent muscle contraction headaches may benefit from a hot shower or moist heat applied to the back of the neck. Cervical collars are sometimes recommended as an aid to good posture. Physical therapy, massage and gentle exercise of the neck may also be helpful.

VASCULAR HEADACHES

Vascular headaches are so named because they are thought to involve abnormal function of the brain's blood vessels or vascular system. These include migraine and its variants as well as headaches due to abnormal stretching of the arterial walls in the cranium as a result of vessel-wall disease.

Migraine

Migraine is an all too common problem today. A recent study suggests that 8.7 million women and 2.6 million men suffer from migraine with moderate to severe disability. Of these, 3.4 million women and 1.1 million men experience one or more attacks per month.[2]

Orthodox medicine holds that the fundamental cause of migraine is unknown. The herbalist, as with most holistically orientated practitioners, can achieve excellent results with migraine by focusing on a number of factors which suggest causal links. Specific herbal remedies can prove exceptionally successful if used in the context of addressing the whole body and environment of the patient.

Although the precise cause of migraine headaches is unknown, a key element is blood flow changes in the brain. People who get migraine headaches appear to have blood vessels that overreact to various triggers. One theory which might explain these changes suggests that the nervous system responds to a trigger by creating a spasm in the nerve-rich arteries at the base of the brain. The spasm closes down or constricts several arteries supplying blood to the brain, including the scalp artery and the carotid or neck arteries. As these arteries constrict, the flow of blood to the brain is reduced. At the same time, blood-clotting particles called platelets clump together, a process which is believed to release a chemical called serotonin. Serotonin acts as a powerful constrictor of arteries, further reducing the blood supply to the brain. Reduced blood flow decreases the brain's supply of oxygen. Symptoms signaling a headache, such as distorted vision or speech, may then result.

Reacting to the reduced oxygen supply, certain arteries within the brain open wider to meet the brain's energy needs. This widening or dilation spreads, finally affecting the neck and scalp arteries. The dilation of these arteries triggers the release of pain-producing substances called prostaglandins from various tissues and blood cells. Chemicals which cause inflammation and swelling and substances which increase sensitivity to pain are also released. The circulation of these chemicals and the dilation of the scalp arteries stimulate the pain-sensitive nerve endings called nociceptors. The result, according to this theory: a throbbing pain in the head.

Migraine attacks commonly take one of two forms. The most common is called migraine without aura (common migraine), accounting for 85 percent of all migraine headaches. These are characterized by episodes of severe, often throbbing pain that may affect only one side of the head, although both sides may be affected. The signature of these headaches is that they are usually, but not always, associated with a feeling of being sick to the stomach or of sensitivity to light, sound or movement of the body. Typically the sufferer wishes to lie down in a dark and quiet room and wait for the storm to pass. Often, those people close to a patient can predict when headache will occur because of changes in the patient's behavior, which may range from depression to exhilaration. If the headache is not relieved early by sleeping it off, it may wax and wane for days, accompanied by appetite loss, nausea or vomiting—hallmarks of the so-called sick headache.

The second most common type is called migraine with aura (classical migraine). The aura of this type of headache, which accounts for most of the remaining 15 percent of migraines, is caused by a disturbance in the nervous system that precedes the headache. Typical disturbances would involve bright flashing lights, black spots, a partial loss of vision or a feeling of pins and needles moving over one limb or one side of the body. These disturbances are usually short-lived, less than one hour for most sufferers, and almost invariably disappear leaving no long-lasting effects.

Other Vascular Headaches[3]

•Toxic headache

After migraine, the most common type of vascular headache is the so-called "toxic" headache experienced during a fever. Pneumonia, flu, measles, mumps and tonsillitis are examples of the diseases that can cause severe toxic vascular headaches.

•Chemical headache

Repeated exposure to nitrite compounds can result in a dull, pounding headache that may be accompanied by a flushed face. Nitrite, which dilates blood vessels, is found in such diverse products as heart medicine and dynamite. Hot dogs and other meats containing sodium nitrite can also cause headaches. Headache can also result from exposure to other poisons, even common household products like insecticides, carbon tetrachloride and lead. Children who eat flakes of lead paint may develop headaches. So may anyone who has contact with lead batteries or lead-glazed pottery. Painters, printmakers and other artists may experience headaches after exposure to art materials that contain chemicals called solvents. Solvents, like benzene, are found in turpentine, spray adhesives, rubber cement and inks.

•**"Chinese restaurant headache"**

This can occur when a susceptible person eats foods prepared with monosodium glutamate (MSG). Soy sauce, meat tenderizer and a variety of packaged foods might contain this chemical, which is used as a flavor-enhancer.

•**Hangover headache**

Jokes are often made about alcohol hangovers, but the headache associated with "the morning after" is no laughing matter. The hangover headache may be reduced by taking honey, which speeds alcohol metabolism, or caffeine, a constrictor of dilated arteries. Caffeine, however, can cause headaches as well as cure them. Heavy coffee drinkers often get headaches when they try to break the caffeine habit.

•**External compression headache**

This refers to the occasional complaint of steady headache provoked by a tight hat or band on the head.

•**"Ice cream headache"**

Such headaches develop in cold weather, after a swim in cold water or after the ingestion of cold food.

•**Benign cough headache**

If a patient suffers head pain brought on by coughing over a long period of time intracranial pathology should be ruled out as a cause. This syndrome may develop in mid-life or later, last several months and spontaneously resolve.

•**Benign exertional headache**

These may be brought on by exercise of any sort; like the external compression headache, more common in those who suffer from migraine. If these headaches continue to interfere with athletic endeavors, they may be prevented by specific therapy for migraine.

•Headache associated with sexual activity

These usually start as a dull diffuse pain and intensify as sexual excitement increases, sometimes becoming very intense at the time of orgasm. Occasionally, patients complain of "postcoital headache" that is intensified when they are upright but is relieved when they recline.

•Drug-induced headache

Headaches are one of the most common side effects to prescription and over-the-counter drugs, making it very difficult to list all potential problem medicines. However those listed below can cause significant headaches.

Drugs That May Cause Headaches

Amyl nitrate
Bromocriptine (Parlodel)
Caffeine
Clonidine (Catapres)
Ergotamine (Ergostat)
Etretinate
Hydralazine (Alazines)
Ibuprofen (Advil)
Indomethacin (Indocin)
Labetalol (Normodyn)
Naproxen (Naprosyn)
Nifedipine (Procardia)
Nitrofurantoin
   (Macrodantin)

Nitroglycerin
Perhexilene (Pexid)
Phenytoin sodium
   (Dilantin)
Propranolol (Inderol)
Sulindac (Clinoril)
Terbutaline (Brethine)
Tetracyclines
Theophylline (Theophyl)
Tolmetin (Tolectin)
Trimethoprim/
   sulfamethoxazole
Warfarin (Coumadin)

Drugs That May Worsen Pre-existing Headaches

Estrogen administered cyclically
Progesterone (Progelan)
Danazol (Danocrine)

Sinus Headaches

In a condition called acute sinusitis, a viral or bacterial infection of the upper respiratory tract spreads to the membrane which lines the sinus cavities. When one or all four of these cavities are filled with bacterial or viral fluid, they become inflamed, causing pain and sometimes headache. The particular cavity affected determines the location of the sinus headache. Chronic sinusitis may be caused by an allergy to such irritants as dust, ragweed, animal hair and smoke.

The sinuses are bony cavities behind, above and at each side of the nose and opening into the nasal cavity. They act as a sound box to give resonance to the voice. Like the nasal passages, the sinuses are lined with mucous membranes, which react to infection by producing mucus. This incapacitates infecting bacteria. Because the openings from the nose into the sinuses are very narrow, they quickly become blocked when the mucous membrane of the nose becomes swollen during a cold, hay fever or catarrh, and then the infection is trapped inside the sinus. Chronic sinusitis may occur if one or more of the drainage passages from the sinuses to the nose becomes blocked. This can cause a dull pain across the face, temples, around the eyes and head.

The herbal approach to these problems can be both indirect and direct. The indirect approach regards upper respiratory disease within the context of the person's health. Sometimes, the overproduction of mucus is an attempt by the body to discharge waste material which is not being properly eliminated by the bowels, kidneys and skin. In such cases, the herbalist may prescribe bitter tonics such as gentian to encourage regular bowel movements, diuretic herbs such as dandelion leaf which encourage kidney elimination of retained fluids and waste materials, or diaphoretic herbs such as yarrow or boneset which stimulate skin elimination.

A direct approach would involve using actively analgesic herbs to kill the pain. There are a number of very effective plants that can do this but they are unfortunately unavailable for general use. It is these very plants that were the original source of the prescription painkillers. The problem with these herbs as well as with the drugs is one of potential dependency.

A diet which reduces mucus production is also essential. In particular, a fruit fast for two or three days can help clear a system clogged and overburdened by toxic wastes. Hot lemon drinks reduce mucus production and so do garlic, onions and horseradish (grate the fresh root into cider vinegar or lemon juice and eat a little each day). Mustard and aromatic herbs like oregano may also be added to the food. Extra zinc and vitamin C will help build up the body's resistance to infection.

Sometimes, emotional factors like suppressed grief can lead to blocked upper respiratory passages. In these cases, a good cry can free this blocked energy and alleviate the problem. Some cases of chronic mucus production are due to allergy.

The herbal approach to sinus headaches is to clear the sinuses rather than simply to kill the pain. Antimicrobial herbs are pivotal in the treatment of this often entrenched condition. These herbs will help the body deal with any infection present and also support the immune system in resisting the development of secondary infection. Remedies known as anticatarrhals will ease the symptomatic discomfort that is characteristic of this problem, also helping the body in the removal of the buildup of mucus in the sinus cavities.

Sinus Headache Formula
- **Goldenrod**
- **Elder flowers**
- **Echinacea**
- **Wild indigo**

Combine equal parts of the tinctures of these herbs and take ½ tsp. of the combination 3 times a day.

A steam inhalant is also an effective technique for treating upper respiratory catarrh and sinusitis. In a bottle, mix 2 Tbs. of compound tincture of benzoin with ½ tsp. eucalyptus oil, 6 drops peppermint oil, 5 drops lavender oil and 5 drops pine oil. Shake well. Put a teaspoonful of this mixture in a bowl with 1 pint boiled water. Cover the head and the bowl with a towel or cloth and inhale. Be sure to keep your eyes closed to avoid irritation.

Certain foods, especially dairy produces and wheat, seem to predispose people toward sinusitis because they provoke excessive formation of mucus. During an acute attack of sinusitis all dairy and wheat-based foods must be excluded for several days, and people who have chronic or repeated attacks are advised to exclude these foods completely for several months, reintroducing them in very small amounts, if at all. Goat's and sheep's milk products are sometimes better tolerated than cow's milk. Acupuncture is a very effective therapy for sinusitis and can be used along with herbal therapy.

Herbal Approaches to Alleviating Headaches

There is an abundance of plants that might be considered "headache" herbs. Unfortunately they don't always work for all people! A representative listing would include the following commonly available remedies:

Chamomile	Peppermint
Dandelion root	Pulsatilla
Elder flower	Rosemary
Feverfew	Rue
Ginger	Skullcap
Lavender	Thyme
Lemon Balm	Valerian
Marjoram	Wood betony

None of these plants are painkillers in the strict sense, that is they do not block the experience of pain. An example of a medicinal plant that does is the opium poppy. The most effective plant painkillers are controlled by law as they can potentially lead to dependency and addiction. Because of that it is often more effective in practice to use indirect pathways. The herbs listed here appear to work by addressing the cause of the pain rather than the experience of pain. Being anti-inflammatory and muscle-relaxing antispasmodic herbs, they alleviate the processes that underlie most muscle contraction and tension headaches.

"NATURAL ASPIRIN"

A large range of plants contain natural "aspirin-type" chemicals called salicylates. It is worth noting that the whole aspirin group of drugs was originally isolated from plant sources. In fact the name aspirin comes from the old botanical genus name for meadowsweet, *Spiraea aspirin*, and salicylate derives from willow's Latin name, *salix*. Those herbs with significant quantities of salicylates have a marked anti-inflammatory effect, without the dangers to the stomach of aspirin itself. In fact meadowsweet, rich in salicylates, can be used to staunch mild stomach hemorrhage even though pharmaceutical salicylates can cause such problems. Other plants rich in such constituents include willow bark, wintergreen, birch, many of the poplars, and black haw.

Salicylates are indeed "aspirin-like" in terms of their chemistry but their properties are subtly different. The main difference is that salicylates do not cross what is known as the blood-brain barrier and so cannot directly effect neurons or block pain transmission. No other body organ is so absolutely dependent on a constant internal environment as is the brain. Other body tissues can withstand the rather small fluctuations in the concentrations of hormones, ions and nutrients that continually occur, particularly after eating or exercising. If the brain were exposed to such chemical changes, uncontrolled neural activity might result. Consequently, neurons are kept separated from blood-borne substances by a so-called blood-brain barrier composed of the least permeable capillaries in the whole body. Only water, glucose, some amino acids and respiratory gases pass easily through the walls of these capillaries.

In practice, then, herbs rich in this group of constituents are most useful in inflammations of muscles, bones and connective tissue caused by conditions such as osteoarthritis or sports injuries. Thus they are of great help in headaches that stem from such causes and are far less helpful in stress or tension headaches.

The analgesic and fever-lowering actions of salicylates are believed to be due to their ability to interfere with the transmission of signals to parts of the hypothalamus, leading to an increase in peripheral blood flow and sweating. Salicylates are also believed to suppress the synthesis of inflammatory prostaglandins, influence arachidonic acid metabolism, increase corticoid levels and inhibit hyaluronidase, thereby reducing inflammation.

Unlike aspirin, willow preparations do not inhibit cyclooxygenase in thrombocytes or the aggregation of platelets, suggesting a different mechanism of action than those associated with salicylates. Because of this, willows and other salicin-containing herbs should not be used as substitutes for aspirin as a preventive protocol against strokes and heart attacks.

ESSENTIAL OILS AND AROMATHERAPY

Aromatherapy, a healing system based on the external application of the essential oils found in aromatic herbs, has much to offer in the relief of headaches. Particularly effective oils are lavender, rosemary, marjoram, chamomile and peppermint, either separately or in combination.

Lavender can be rubbed on the temples or made into a

cold compress and applied to the temples, forehead or the back of the neck. Equal parts of lavender and peppermint may be even more effective, for lavender has the ability to enhance the action of other oils when it is used in blends.

If the headache is caused by catarrh or sinus infection, inhalations with lavender, peppermint, rosemary or eucalyptus will usually be very effective in both relieving the headache and clearing the congestion that is causing it. All these oils are antiseptic and will combat the nasal infection and give immediate relief of symptoms.

The following descriptions include oils that are not specific for headaches but will be found useful in certain causes of headaches. The best way to use this list is to first have an insight into the cause of a specific headache, for example is it related to stress, worry, food sensitivities, etc.? On this basis the relevant essential oil can be then identified to address the cause rather than the result.

Essential Oil	Properties
Bergamot	Antidepressant, antiparasitic, anti-inflammatory, antiseptic. Enhances immunity, treats genital, urinary, mouth and throat infections, flu, herpes, shingles and chicken pox; aids digestion. It is a traditional Italian folk medicine for fever and intestinal worms.
Chamomile	Anti-inflammatory, antiallergenic, digestive, relaxant, antidepressant. Used to treat the inflammation of sore muscles, sprains, tendons and joints as well as headaches, diarrhea, digestive tract ulcers, asthma and allergies. It helps reduce indigestion, PMS, menstrual pain, liver damage and children's hyperactivity. It also destroys various types of in-

testinal worms and improves immune system activity.

Clary sage — Antidepressant, relaxant, eases muscle and nervous tension, pain, menstrual cramps, PMS and menopause problems such as hot flashes. It also stimulates adrenals and is a European remedy for sore throat. Used to treat postpartum depression and stress-related conditions.

Cypress — Astringent, stimulating to circulation, antiseptic. Treats low blood pressure, poor circulation, varicose veins and hemorrhoids. It alleviates laryngitis, spasmodic coughing, lung congestion, urinary problems and cellulite. It is a deodorant and reduces excessive fluids in the body associated with conditions such as diarrhea and runny nose.

Eucalyptus — Decongestant, antiviral, antibacterial, stimulant. Treats sinus and throat infection, fever, flu, chicken pox and herpes. It is specific for thin mucus with chills and lack of thirst.

Geranium — Balancing to mind and body, antifungal, anti-inflammatory. A light adrenal stimulant and hormonal normalizer; treats PMS, menopause, fluid retention, breast engorgement and sterility.

Helichrysum — Antidepressant, treats infection and inflammation of chronic cough, bronchitis, fever, muscle pain, arthritis, phlebitis and liver problems and counters allergic reactions such as asthma. Used to lift depression, lethargy, nervous exhaustion and stress.

Lavender
Excellent first-aid oil; antiviral, antibacterial, boosts immunity, antidepressant, anti-inflammatory, antispasmodic. Used to treat lung, sinus and vaginal infections, including *candida*. An excellent treatment for laryngitis and asthma. It relieves muscle pain, headaches, insect bites, cystitis and other inflammation. It also treats digestive disturbances, including colic.

Marjoram
Antispasmodic, anti-inflammatory, antiseptic. A strong sedative, eases muscle spasms, tics, menstrual cramps, headaches (especially migraines) and stiff joints. Treats spasmodic coughs, colds, flu, laryngitis and hypertension and is a light laxative. Also helps normalize blood pressure.

Neroli
Antidepressant, aphrodisiac. Neroli treats diarrhea and circulation problems such as hemorrhoids and high blood pressure. Used to counter emotional shock, mental confusion, nervous strain, anxiety, fear and lack of confidence.

Peppermint
Digestive; clears sinuses, antiseptic, decongestant, stimulant. Peppermint alleviates digestive tract spasms, indigestion, nausea, ulcers and irritable bowel syndrome, and helps destroy bacteria, viruses and parasites in the digestive tract. It also clears sinus and lung congestion and is used to treat muscle spasms and inflammation.

Rosemary
Stimulating to circulation, relieves pain, decongestant, improves circulation. One

of the best stimulants, it also lowers cholesterol, eases muscle and rheumatism pains and treats lung congestion, sore throat and canker sores. It stimulates the nervous system, motor nerves, adrenals and a sluggish gallbladder. It is often used in penetrating liniments.

Tea tree   Antifungal, antiyeast, antibacterial. A good immune system tonic which fights lung, genital, urinary, vaginal, sinus and mouth infections. It counters fungal infections and viral infections such as herpes, shingles, chicken pox, *candida*, thrush and flu.

Ylang-ylang   Strong sedative, antispasmodic. Helps to lower blood pressure, tempers depression, fear, anger, aphrodisiac in small doses. High concentration can produce headaches or nausea.

Essential oils can have an impact not only on physical issues such as muscle tension and inflammation but also on emotional states. The following summary of the psychological indications for the essential oils comes from an excellent and comprehensive guide entitled *Aromatherapy* by Kathi Keville and Mindy Green.

Emotion	Oils
Anger	Basil, Chamomile, Cinnamon, Coriander, Frankincense, Geranium, Hyssop, Jasmine, Lavender, Melissa, Neroli, Pine, Rose, Rosewood, Ylang-ylang.
Anxiety	Basil, Benzoin, Bergamot, Camphor, Cardamom, Chamomile, Cypress, Fennel, Frankincense, Geranium, Jasmine,

	Juniper, Lavender, Marjoram, Melissa, Nutmeg, Patchouli, Petitgrain, Peppermint, Pine, Rose, Rosemary, Rosewood, Sandalwood, Ylang-ylang.
Apathy	Geranium, Jasmine, Neroli, Patchouli, Peppermint, Pine, Rose, Rosemary, Rosewood, Sage.
Confusion	Basil, Camphor, Cardamom, Cedar, Cinnamon, Cypress, Frankincense, Helichrysum, Hyssop, Jasmine, Lavender, Lemon, Marjoram, Neroli, Patchouli, Peppermint, Sandalwood.
Depression	Basil, Bergamot, Chamomile, Clary sage, Coriander, Frankincense, Geranium, Helichrysum, Lavender, Lemon neroli, Patchouli, Petitgrain, Peppermint, Pine, Rose, Rosewood, Sandalwood, Vetivert, Ylang-ylang.
Fear	Basil, Chamomile, Coriander, Fennel, Hyssop, Jasmine, Melissa, Neroli, Orange, Rose, Thyme.
Forgetfulness	Basil, Bay, Coriander, Melissa, Rosemary, Ylang-ylang.
Grief	Cypress, Hyssop, Jasmine, Marjoram, Rose, Rosemary, Sage.
Hypersensitivity	Cedar, Chamomile, Clary sage, Eucalyptus, Geranium, Hyssop, Juniper, Lavender, Marjoram, Myrrh, Neroli, Patchouli, Rose, Ylang-ylang.
Impatience	Bergamot, Camphor, Chamomile, Fennel, Frankincense, Jasmine, Lavender, Marjoram, Myrrh, Rose.
Instability	Anise, Benzoin, Bergamot, Camphor, Chamomile, Cypress, Geranium, Helichrysum, Hyssop, Lavender, Lemon,

	Marjoram, Myrrh, Rosemary, Sandalwood, Thyme.
Insomnia	Bergamot, Chamomile, Cypress, Frankincense, Geranium, Jasmine, Lavender, Lemon, Marjoram, Melissa, Myrrh, Neroli, Nutmeg, Patchouli, Petitgrain, Rose, Sage, Sandalwood, Ylang-ylang.
Melancholy	Benzoin, Frankincense, Lavender, Marjoram, Melissa, Peppermint, Rose, Rosemary, Rosewood, Sandalwood, Thyme.
Panic/Shock	Bay, Camphor, Chamomile, Clary Sage, Coriander, Eucalyptus, Jasmine, Lavender, Melissa, Orange, Patchouli, Petitgrain, Peppermint, Rosewood, Vetivert, Ylang-ylang.
Stress	Anise, Basil, Bay, Bergamot, Cardamom, Chamomile, Clary sage, Eucalyptus, Fennel, Frankincense, Helichrysum, Juniper, Lavender, Lemon, Marjoram, Neroli, Nutmeg, Orange, Peppermint, Rose, Rosewood, Sage, Sandalwood, Thyme, Ylang-ylang.
Irritability	Cedar, Clary sage, Cinnamon, Cypress, Melissa, Neroli, Orange, Patchouli.

There are a range of ways to use essential oils. The dilutions given below are for adults, so halve them for children, and use them at quarter strength for infants. Be careful with essential oils, always dilute them, and *never* use them internally.

Massage oils. Always dilute oils before applying them to the skin. Use a carrier oil such as sweet almond oil, jojoba oil or any other pure, unblended vegetable oil. Do not use mineral oils, unlike vegetable oils, they will not be absorbed by the skin. 3-5 drops of essential oils to 2 tsp. of a carrier oil is usually appropriate.

Baths. Add up to 5 drops of pure essential oil to a bath full of warm water. Float the oil on the surface and stir with your hand before relaxing in the bath for 10-15 minutes. For a hand or foot soak use 2-3 drops in a bowl of warm water. Add 20-40 drops to 1 cup of bath salts.

Inhalation. Add 2-5 drops of essential oil to a bowl of hot water, cover your head with a towel and inhale the fragrant steam or put 1-2 drops directly onto a cotton ball for a convenient way to inhale the aroma.

Treatments for Headaches

Despite taking preventive measures, almost everyone gets a headache sometimes. Here are some suggestions for immediate headache relief. Ice packs are among the most effective nondrug treatments. The earlier an ice pack is used to treat a headache, the better. Besides applying it to the painful area, try placing it on the back of the neck, forehead and temples.

- **For tension headache.** Try heat or ice packs, a hot shower and rest. Take a break from a stressful situation.
- **For migraine.** Sleep. Take a nap in a dark, quiet room. Press an ice pack to the back of your neck and apply gentle pressure to painful scalp areas.

Over the long term try these steps:

- Control triggers. See page 35
- Keep a headache calendar to help identify those factors that cause your headaches so you can avoid them.
- Limit the use of pain relievers.
- If you smoke, quit. Smoking may bring on either a migraine or a cluster headache and increase its intensity.
- Manage stress. Exercise regularly. However, if physical activity brings on a migraine, make sure you first warm up slowly.

Sometimes depression, anxiety or other kinds of emotional problems are associated with chronic and severe headaches. In fact headaches can be an important marker for depression.[4] You may need to focus more on treating the entity of depression than on treating the symptom of headache. Consider individual or family counseling to help minimize the impact of emotional problems on your headaches. Counseling may also help reduce the negative effects your headaches may have on your family. You might also join a headache support group.

TREATMENT OF TENSION HEADACHES

Herbal medicine has the most to contribute in the alleviation of tension headaches because it helps to ease anxiety and serves as a component of stress management programs. This is discussed in depth in my companion volume, *Herbs to Relieve Stress.*

If a period of stress is predictably about to occur, it can be prepared for ahead of time, as herbs, diet and lifestyle changes will minimize the impact. Nervine relaxants can be used regularly as gentle soothing remedies. Those listed below are examples. These herbs can be taken as teas or cold drinks, infused in massage oil or used in relaxing footbaths or full baths.

Chamomile	Mugwort
Lavender	Oats
Lemon Balm	Skullcap
Linden blossom	Vervain

A daily supplement of the B-complex vitamins and vitamin C is also helpful. As well as responding to stress in a healthy way by using herbs and improving the diet, you can try to soften the impact of the various stressors. It helps to re-evaluate choices. Ask yourself these questions:

- Are you doing what you really want to do?
- If not, what would you rather be doing?

Give yourself permission to ask some questions about yourself and your lifestyle without censoring any of the answers that may come up. After pinpointing inner motivations, choices can be made about what you want to do about them. Relaxation exercises and an honest re-evaluation of both lifestyle and life goals are invaluable.

One possible prescription for stress and tension-related headaches is as follows:

Tension Headache Formula I

Skullcap	2 parts
Valerian	2 parts
Oats	1 part

As a tincture, take ½ tsp. of this mixture 3 times a day. As a tea, infuse 2 tsp. dried mixture in a cup of boiling water for 10-15 minutes and drink 3 times a day.

Stress reactions often have accompanying physical symptoms, so here is an example of one possible prescription for acute stress associated with indigestion and palpitations:

Tension Headache Formula II

Skullcap	2 parts
Valerian	2 parts
Motherwort	1 part
Chamomile	1 part
Mugwort	1 part

As a tincture, take 1 tsp. of this mixture 3 times a day. As a tea infuse 2 tsp. dried mixture in 1 cup boiling water for 10-15 minutes and drink 3 times a day.

Motherwort supports the relaxing of the other nervines

but also has a specific calming impact upon heart palpitations.

In their exceptional book, authors Kathi Keville and Mindy Green recommend the following combinations for headache relief[5]:

Massage or Bath Oil Formula
   3 drops **lavender**
   3 drops **neroli**
   2 drops **marjoram**
   2 drops **ylang-ylang**
   1 drop **chamomile**
   2 drops **clary sage**
   1 oz. carrier oil

Bath Oil Formula
   3 drops **chamomile** oil
   3 drops **lavender** oil
   2 drops **marjoram** oil
   2 drops **thyme** oil
   1 drop **coriander** oil

Disperse the oils in a bathtub filled with warm water. Soak in the bath for 20 to 30 minutes. Repeat as necessary.

Neuralgia, or nerve pain, is best remedied by treating the cause, although essential oils do alleviate the pain, especially when used in conjunction with massage.

Massage Oil Formula for Neuralgia
   5 drops **helichrysum**
   3 drops **chamomile**
   2 drops **marjoram**
   2 drops **lavender**
   1 ounce carrier oil
Combine ingredients and use for massage.

Chamomile Muscle-relaxing Compresses

Hot chamomile compresses work well for the relaxation of painful tense muscles. Prepare a strong infusion with 1 full cup of chamomile flowers and 2 quarts of boiling water; cover with a lid and allow to steep for about 10 minutes, then strain off through a sieve. Dip one cloth into the infusion, wring it out and place it as hot as tolerable on the back, shoulders and neck. Soak the other cloth in the hot infusion, wring it out, and place it on top of the first one. Now turn both cloths over so that the fresh hot compress is against the patient's skin. Remove the upper towel and soak it in the mixture. Repeat the procedure 10 to 20 times until there is a sense of relaxation and loss of tension.

TREATMENT OF MIGRAINE

It would be claiming far too much to say that herbal medicine can cure migraine. However, when selected with care, certain plants have much to offer in the amelioration and control of this distressing problem. By far the most important is a common roadside plant called feverfew.

Feverfew (*Tanacetum parthenium*) is commonly used in European herbal medicine as a specific remedy for the treatment of migraine. It is also the best example of a remedy long known to medical herbalists that has also recently been accepted and used by allopathic medicine.[6] It has been used throughout recorded medical history as a bitter tonic and remedy for severe headaches. Through wide media coverage in recent years, the herb has gained a well-deserved reputation as a "cure" for migraine. Clinicians at the London Migraine Clinic observed that patients were reporting marked improvements when they took the herb. Thankfully, these doctors had the inquiring and open minds of true scientists and so started their own investigations into the claims for feverfew. Clinical observations were soon reported in peer-reviewed medical journals.

The first double-blind study was done at the London Migraine Clinic, using patients who reported being helped by feverfew.[7] Seventeen patients who regularly ate fresh leaves of feverfew daily to prevent migraine were invited to participate in a double-blind, placebo-controlled trial of the herb. Of these, eight patients received capsules containing freeze-dried feverfew powder and nine, a placebo. Those patients who received the placebo (and as a result stopped using feverfew) had a significant increase in the frequency and severity of headaches, nausea and vomiting during the six months of the study as well as the re-emergence of untoward effects during the early months of treatment. The group given capsules of feverfew, on the other hand, showed no change in the lack of symptoms of migraine, providing clear evidence that feverfew can prevent attacks of migraine. Two patients in the placebo group who had been in complete remission during self-treatment with feverfew leaves developed a recurrence of incapacitating migraine and had to withdraw from the study. The resumption of self-treatment led to renewed remission of symptoms in both patients. This led the researchers to strongly suggest the use of feverfew for all migraine sufferers.

Another double-blind study was performed at the University of Nottingham. The results of the study clearly demonstrated that feverfew was effective in reducing the number and severity of migraine attacks and confirmed that a daily intake of feverfew prophylactically prevents attacks of migraine.[8]

Follow-up studies to clinical results have shown feverfew works in the treatment and prevention of migraine headaches by inhibiting the release of blood vessel-dilating substances from platelets, inhibiting the production of inflammatory substances and re-establishing proper blood vessel tone.

The effectiveness of feverfew is dependent upon adequate levels of parthenolide, the active ingredient. The preparations used in the clinical trials had a parthenolide content of 0.2 percent. The dosage of feverfew used in the London Migraine Clinic study was one capsule containing 25 mg of the freeze-dried pulverized leaves twice daily. In the Nottingham study, it was one capsule containing 82 mg of dried powdered leaves once daily. While these low dosages may be effective in preventing an attack, a higher dose (1 to 2 grams) is necessary during an acute attack. Feverfew is extremely well-tolerated and no serious side effects have been reported. However, chewing the leaves can result in small ulcerations in the mouth and swelling of the lips and tongue. This condition occurs in about 10 percent of users.

The venerable English herbalists Gerard and Culpepper would not have been surprised at all at these findings. It is a pity that the patients given the placebo had to go through the renewed migraine attacks to demonstrate something already well-known to herbalists and the patients themselves.

Pharmacologists are putting great attention on the humble "weed," feverfew, in the search for a new class of effective and profitable antimigraine and analgesic drugs. Since the simple dried or fresh leaf of feverfew is such an excellent formulation for preventing migraine why don't doctors prescribe it? The reasons are social, political and economic as well as medical. Since the plant is grown by nature free of charge and is not patentable, there is no profit in it for the pharmaceutical industry. Moreover, most of the information passed on to doctors is generated by that industry.

Following the clinical clues, pharmacologists are finding active components in the plant. Part of the herb's action appears to be its ability to inhibit secretion of the granular contents from platelets and neutrophils in the blood. This may be relevant to the therapeutic value of feverfew in migraine and other conditions such as osteoarthritis.

The five main compounds that were identified as having this activity were parthenolide, 3-beta-hydroxy-parthenolide, secotanapartholide-A, canin and artecanin, all of which are sesquiterpene lactones.[9] The researchers say that it is very likely that these and other sesquiterpene lactones inhibit prostaglandins and histamine released during the inflammatory process, thereby preventing spasms of the blood vessels in the head that trigger migraine attacks.[10,11] Other studies indicate that feverfew inhibits interactions of human platelets and polymorphonuclear leukocytes with collagen substrates.[12] It has been suggested that its medicinal properties are related to the inhibition of secretory activity.

As with all such impressive research findings that isolate "active" ingredients, it is important not to lose sight of the importance of the whole plant activity. Considerable differences in the parthenolide content of feverfew have been observed in plants from different geographical localities.[13] Similarly, commercial preparations of dried feverfew usually contain varying amounts of the active principle.[14] For this reason standardized preparations are often used today. A daily dosage of 125 mg of a dried feverfew leaf preparation from *Tanacetum parthenium*, containing at least 0.2 percent parthenolide, is considered appropriate for the treatment and prevention of migraines. This equates to approximately 250 mcg of parthenolide daily.

Feverfew is a long-term treatment, not an immediate cure for a migraine attack. Clinical experience suggests that four to six weeks are usually required to note an initial response. However, average duration of use will vary among migraine patients. Success should be measured by decreased frequency, severity and duration of migraine attacks. Don't use feverfew if you are pregnant or breast-feeding. If you are already taking prescription medications for migraines, consult a healthcare professional before using feverfew.

Some people find that regular use of feverfew is enough to control or even clear their migraines. However, for others, additional herbal support may also be in order. Ginkgo offers some very relevant properties mainly due to its ability to tone the blood vessel walls as well as reduce the tendency for platelet clumping to occur. Ginkgo extract standardized to 24 percent flavone glycosides is recommended at a dose of 120 mg daily in two to three divided doses.

Many phytotherapists in Britain focus upon supporting the liver in migraine treatments. As an example consider the following mixture suggested by Mrs. Nalda Gosling F.N.I.M.H., one of Britain's most respected herbal clinicians.

Mrs. Gosling's Formula for Migraine

Mix equal parts of the following dried herbs:

Motherwort	**Centaury**
Vervain	**Wild carrot**
Dandelion root	

Simmer ¾ oz. of this mixture for 15 minutes in 2 cups of water. Strain. Drink 4-6 oz. of this tea 3 times a day.

European Folk Remedy for Migraine

Make a tea mixture of the following dried herbs:
2 parts **rosemary**
2 parts **peppermint**

2 parts **lemon balm**
1 part **sweet violet**
1 part **feverfew**

Steep 1 tsp. of this mixture in 1 cup of boiling water for 10-15 minutes. Strain and drink 3 times a day.

This tea has a very fine flavor and can be enjoyed daily. Homeopathy and traditional herbalism agree that sweet violet, which hides from the sun and loves the shade, can be of help to migraine patients who cannot tolerate bright sunlight and seek darkness and shade.

Cooling Compress for Migraine

1 quart ice-cold water
2 drops **peppermint** oil
1 drop **ginger** oil
1 drop **marjoram** oil

Pour the water into a two-quart glass bowl and add the essential oils. Soak a clean cloth in the water and apply it to your head, forehead or neck at the first sign of a developing migraine. Avoid letting the compress come into contact with your eyes. Apply an ice pack over the compress to keep it cold.

MIGRAINE TRIGGERS AND CONTRIBUTING FACTORS

Early signs of a headache and whatever sets it off are critical to notice. These signs may be actual beginnings of the headache or physical events that almost invariably lead to a headache. Catching the very early signs of a headache, perhaps even before pain begins but certainly before it becomes severe, can give you important clues to controlling a headache. These early signs may be symptoms of aura, aching muscles, cold hands, a general sense of tension or any number of other indications.

A **trigger** for headache pain may be almost anything in one's lifestyle or environment. Triggers don't cause the pain; rather, they activate an already existing chemical mechanism in the brain. For example, does drinking red wine lead to a headache within a few hours? If so, we could call red wine a trigger.

Most people's headaches are triggered not by one factor but by the interaction of several. In general, the more triggers present at any given time, the more likely a headache is to follow. In one study, migraine patients reported an average of five triggers. This has important ramifications as it demands that triggers be observed systematically over time and that all be considered.

Factors that increase one's vulnerability to headache, but do not immediately lead to one, are called contributing or contextual factors. Such factors create a context in which a headache is more likely to be set off by triggers. Some people can develop migraine not only during a period of stress but also afterwards, when their vascular systems are still reacting. Migraines that wake people in the middle of the night are also believed to result from a delayed reaction to stress.

General "toxicity," that is, any tendency to constipation, liver problems or general congestion will be a marked trigger in some individuals. Structural, cranial and spinal misalignments may also be involved, as may poor posture, even when not associated with overt skeletal problems.

Common headache triggers include:

- **Stress.** Particularly for chronic tension headaches or migraine, stress can be a powerful trigger. Stress can come from major life events such as a divorce or moving, but everyday hassles like commuting or a demanding boss can have an even bigger effect.

- **Emotions.** Common negative emotions such as depression, anxiety, a sense of letdown, frustration as well as positive pleasant excitement can trigger headaches.
- **Muscle tension.** Almost all individuals with chronic headache have some degree of muscle irritation at the upper back, neck and face. The muscle irritation is most often associated with chronic but subtle muscle tension, nothing very dramatic but going on regularly day after day. This is true for both migraine and tension-type headaches. Muscle irritation should be considered a trigger of headache pain. The type of pain triggered reflects a variety of factors, not the least of which is the type of headache to which an individual is prone. Muscle irritation can produce local pain, pain around the site of the muscle irritation, or it can refer pain to sites away from the irritated muscle. For example, muscle irritation at the back of the neck may be felt as severe pain at the temple on the same side of the head. This is called referred pain.

  Chronic muscle tension may arise from a variety of causes—regular poor posture, repeated muscle strain or overuse, tightening up under stress, mannerisms such as frowning or grinding the teeth, or even bracing against headache pain itself. Eventually this tension may lead to very tender muscles, aching with normal movement, stiffness from being in one position for a long time, pain when lying in bed for a prolonged period or even restriction in the mobility of the neck or jaw.

- **Diet.** Between 8 and 25 percent of people with migraine can point to a particular food as a source of their attacks. See next page.
- **Change in the weather, seasons, altitude or time zones.**

- **Change in sleep patterns and meal times.** Both too little or too much sleep can act as triggers.
- **Hormone levels.** The normal fluctuations in hormone levels during the menstrual cycle or pregnancy, or from estrogen replacement therapy can be potent triggers. Oral contraceptives also can worsen migraine. Please see Women and Migraine, page 43 for more details.
- **Sensory irritants,** such as glaring or flickering lights or unusual odors.
- **Polluted air** or stuffy rooms.
- **Smoking.** Suffering from chronic headache is one more good reason to quit smoking. Smoking seems to be a negative factor for those with chronic pain conditions in general. The way in which smoking tobacco might be associated with exacerbation of pain conditions is not known with certainty, but there are many possible routes, and none of them is good for the health. Smoking can cause headaches as nicotine constricts the blood vessels while inhaled carbon monoxide overly expands them, thus creating a condition which often triggers migraines and cluster headaches.
- **Blood Clotting.** Another cause of headaches is blood clotting, also known as platelet aggregation. Clotting creates constriction of the arteries, which results in inadequate blood supply to the brain. This is then followed by a rebound dilation of the blood vessels, leading to headaches.

FOODS THAT CAN TRIGGER HEADACHES

Foods precipitate migraine attacks in many people, not only due to allergies, but also because these foods contain compounds known as "vasoactive amines," which can trigger migraines by causing blood vessels to expand. Many migraine sufferers have been found to have significantly lower levels of a platelet enzyme that normally breaks down these natural dietary components. Since red wine contains substances that are potent inhibitors of this enzyme, it often triggers migraines in these individuals, especially if consumed along with high vasoactive-amine foods like cheese. Alcohol, especially red wine and beer, are among the most likely alcoholic beverages to cause problems. Congeners, the substances that give alcohol its distinguishing characteristics, may trigger migraines along with the alcohol itself.

The naturally occurring amino acid, tyramine, found in foods such as aged cheeses, Chianti wine and pickled herring, affects several mechanisms known to be involved with migraine. Chocolate may be another trigger. But it's not clear whether chocolate causes migraine or whether a sudden craving for chocolate is caused by an impending migraine.

Caffeine can cause headaches by increasing the body's craving for it. When blood levels of caffeine drop, symptoms of withdrawal, including headache, may set in. That's why heavy coffee drinkers experience "morning headache" until they have that first cup of coffee. Headaches related to caffeine involve a dull, throbbing pain on both sides of the head and are generally not as intense as migraine headaches. Once the body rids itself of the caffeine's effects, the headaches will disappear on their own. People who suffer from caffeine headaches are often unaware of the cause, however, and so they do not avoid caffeine, causing the headaches to recur. Food additives, such as sodium nitrite in hot dogs and luncheon meats or monosodium glutamate in many processed foods, may also trigger migraine in some people.

The following foods are known to commonly trigger headaches in sensitive people:

- Red or white wine.
- Other alcoholic beverages.
- Refined sugar products, e.g., sodas and candy.
- Dried fruit.
- Artificial additives, colorings and preservatives, e.g., aspartame (NutraSweet).
- Nuts.
- Onions.
- Herring.
- Chocolate.
- Peanut butter.
- Chicken livers.
- Dairy products, especially sour cream and yogurt.
- Vinegar (except white vinegar).
- Bananas (no more than half a banana per day may be tolerated).
- Anything that is fermented, pickled or marinated.
- Pods of broad beans (lima, navy, pinto, garbanzo and pea).
- Any foods containing large amounts of monosodium glutamate (MSG).
- Caffeine: tea, coffee and cola beverages.
- Citrus fruit (one serving per day may be tolerated).
- Processed meats such as bologna, salami, sausage, pepperoni, hot dogs and ham.
- Hot fresh breads, raised coffee cakes and raised doughnuts (may be tolerated if cool).
- Ripened cheeses such as cheddar, Emmenthaler, Gruyere, Stilton, brie and camembert.

GENERAL DIETARY GUIDELINES

- Eat smaller and more frequent meals.
- Reduce fat intake.

- Reduce caffeine (coffee, tea, cola, chocolate).
- Reduce salt.
- Increase complex carbohydrates, such as peas, rice, squash, beans, corn, potatoes.
- Increase potassium-rich foods such as potatoes, asparagus, celery, apricots, grapes, carrots, broccoli, Brussels sprouts, cauliflower, noncitrus fruits.
- Increase magnesium-rich foods such as dark green vegetables, legumes, whole grains.
- Limit alcohol intake.
- Limit sweets.
- Consider taking the following supplements:
  Magnesium—200 to 300 mg twice daily.
  MaxEPA (fish oil)—3 to 4 grams daily with meals.[15]

SELF-MASSAGE FOR HEADACHES

The following self-massage can provide relief from headache pain. Sit comfortably in a chair, taking care to breathe freely through the diaphragm. Cradle the back of your neck with your hand and squeeze gently, slowly rolling your head from side to side. Release for a few moments, then again squeeze your neck, slightly increasing the pressure. Repeat squeezing and releasing 20 times. Next, using your fingertips, press into any areas in your neck and shoulders that are sore or tender, moving your arms and shoulders in a gentle, rhythmic motion. Continue this for several minutes, until your headache fades.

Doing this massage periodically throughout the day will often prevent headaches from reoccurring. They can also be performed by a partner. As you seat yourself, have your partner stand behind you and follow the above instructions.

A Progressive Relaxation Exercise

The following exercise is one headache sufferers can use to learn how to relax and relieve the stress of muscle tension.

Lie down or lean back in a comfortable chair in a quiet room with subdued light. Take 10 slow, deep breaths, taking a little longer to breathe out than you take to breathe in. The ideal timing is a two-second full inhalation followed by a slow, controlled four- or five-second exhalation. This starts the relaxation process.

Beginning with the feet, clench the toes tightly for a few seconds, then release. Then tighten the muscles of the leg, and relax. Repeat this process for the rest of the body: buttocks, back, abdomen, hands, arms, shoulders, neck, jaw, eyes and finally the muscles of the face. Next, yawn several times, then squeeze the eyes open and shut, taking another 10 deep breaths. Notice how much more relaxed you are. Continue breathing, allowing yourself to relax even more. Then resume your regular activities.

Hydrotherapy

Hydrotherapy is another method for treating headaches without drugs. Hot baths, saunas, heat lamps and steam baths all reduce tension by increasing blood circulation. A migraine headache, for instance, can sometimes be stopped with the combination of a hot shower followed quickly by an ice-cold one. Hot water may at first increase the migraine pain by temporarily dilating blood vessels, but this paves the way for fast relief when the vessels are constricted by the cold shower.

WOMEN AND MIGRAINE

Migraine is more common in adult women than in men. Both sexes may develop migraine in infancy, but most often the disorder begins between the ages of 5 and 35. The relationship between female sex hormones and migraine is unclear, but the association of migraine with menstrual flow seems to arise from the fluctuations in hormonal levels, especially estrogen, rather than from too much or too little of any particular hormone. Some women suffer from "menstrual migraine" around the time of their menstrual period, but the headaches may disappear during pregnancy. Many women trace the onset of their severe headaches to puberty while others develop migraine for the first time when they are pregnant. Still others are first affected after menopause.

The effect of oral contraceptives on headaches is perplexing. Some migrainous women who take birth control pills experience more frequent and severe attacks. However, a small percentage of women have fewer and less severe migraine headaches when they take birth control pills. Women who normally do not suffer from headaches may develop migraines as a side effect when they use oral contraceptives.

The choice of herbs goes beyond the use of feverfew here as the underlying hormonal issues need to be addressed. Remedies that facilitate hormone balancing should always be included, with chasteberry, also called vitex, the most directly relevant.

The first mixture for menstrually related migraine diminishes the symptoms of PMS, thus easing this headache trigger, while the second is the core treatment to be used on a daily basis.

Hormonal Migraine Formula #1

Skullcap	2 parts
Valerian	1 part

Dandelion   1 part

Mix the tinctures together. Take 1 tsp. as needed to alleviate symptoms.

Hormonal Migraine Formula #2

Vitex   2 parts
Feverfew   1 part

Mix the tinctures together. Take 1 tsp. once a day through the month.

The dosage of Formula #1 may be increased until the desired relief is experienced. The dosage regime may be altered as necessary, varying time of day and quantity of dose to suit individual needs. For example, one may take the whole dose first thing in the morning or take smaller amounts at frequent intervals throughout the day.

Herbalists have developed many approaches to migraine, reflecting the diversity of people and their response to herbs. Here is an example from a modern woman herbalist, Deb Soule:[16]

Be as kind and patient with yourself as possible. Migraines usually take a few months or even longer to decrease in severity. The following herbs help to ease a migraine headache. Take as tea or tincture whenever you feel a migraine or regular headache coming on.

Deb Soule's Migraine Formula

Feverfew	3 parts
Lemon balm	1 part
Passionflower	½ part
Rosemary	1 part
Basil	1 part
Ginkgo leaf	2 parts

Dose and use: Pour 1 quart of hot steaming water over 6 Tbs. of herbs and steep, covered, 5 to 15 minutes. Drink

½ cup every hour until symptoms subside. The herbs can also be taken as a tincture, 4 to 6 times a day, 30 to 60 drops each time.

A safe and effective tea that can achieve dramatic results in balancing female hormonal swings if used regularly is this mixture formulated by California herbalist Diana DeLuca:

Diana Deluca's Hormone Balancing Formula

Vitex berries, crushed	3 parts
Ginger root	1 part
Dandelion root	1 part
Licorice root	1 part
Red raspberry leaf	1 part

Make a decoction from this mixture (see page 72) and drink daily.

In European herbalism, vitex and St. John's wort are used extensively for easing the symptomatic discomfort that may accompany the menopausal transition. St. John's wort has a role in lessening any depression that might occur. Both herbs will combine well with feverfew to gradually alleviate menopausal symptoms.[17]

Menopausal Formula
    Vitex
    St. John's wort
Mix equal parts of these tinctures. Take ½ tsp. of the combination 3 times a day.

If headaches occur frequently during menopause, along with other typical symptoms, try a tea blend of equal parts of St. John's wort, balm, skullcap and passionflower.

Materia Medica

number of medicinal plants are described here that are not specific for headaches but will be found useful in certain causes of headaches. The best way to use this information is to first have an insight into the cause of your specific headache. Ideally this will come from a skilled diagnostician who has assessed your general health as well as the type of headache you have.

The herbs listed each have a spectrum of actions and a range of specific indications making them relevant for treatments for one or other of the causes of headaches. For example, if the headache is sinus-based, herbs such as golden rod or eyebright will prove efficacious, whereas if it is related to anxiety, then skullcap or kava kava will be more appropriate. On this basis the relevant herb or herbs can be then identified to address the cause rather than the symptoms of the resulting headache.

BLACK COHOSH   *Cimicifuga racemosa*
Part used: Root and rhizome; dried, not fresh.
Actions: Emmenagogue, antispasmodic, nervine, hypotensive.
Indications: Black cohosh offers a valuable combination of actions that makes it uniquely useful in painful cramping conditions of the female reproductive system. It may be used in cases of painful or delayed menstruation and

ovarian cramps. It is also active in the treatment of rheumatic, muscular and neurological pain. It is useful in sciatica and neuralgia. As a relaxing nervine it may be used in many situations where such an agent is needed. It has been found beneficial in cases of tinnitus.

Preparations & dosage: *Decoction:* Pour a cup of water onto ½ to 1 tsp. of the dried root and bring to boil. Let it simmer for 10 to 15 minutes. Strain. Drink 3 times a day. *Tincture:* Take ¼ tsp. of the tincture 3 times a day.

BLACK HAW   *Viburnum prunifolium*
Part used: Dried bark of root, stem or trunk.

Actions: Antispasmodic, nervine, hypotensive, astringent.

Indications: Black haw has a very similar use to crampbark, to which it is closely related. It is a powerful relaxant of the uterus and is used for dysmenorrhea and false labor pains as well as for threatened miscarriage. Its relaxant and sedative actions explain its power in reducing blood pressure in hypertension, which happens through a relaxation of the peripheral blood vessels. It may be used as an antispasmodic in the treatment of asthma.

Preparations & dosage: *Decoction:* Put 2 tsp. of the dried bark in 1 cup of water, bring to the boil and simmer for 10 minutes: Strain. Drink 3 times a day. *Tincture:* Take 1-2 tsp. of the tincture 3 times a day.

BONESET   *Eupatorium perfoliatum*
Part used: Dried aerial parts.

Actions: Diaphoretic, bitter, laxative, tonic, antispasmodic, carminative, astringent.

Indications: Boneset is one the best remedies for the relief of the associated symptoms that accompany influenza. It will speedily relieve the aches and pains as well as aid the body in dealing with any fever that is present. Boneset may also be used to help clear the upper respiratory tract of mucus congestion. Its mild aperient activity will ease constipation. It may safely be used in any fever and also as a general cleansing agent. It may provide symptomatic aid in the treatment of muscular rheumatism.

Combinations: In the treatment of influenza it may be combined with yarrow, elder flowers, cayenne or ginger, with pleurisy root and elecampane in bronchial conditions.

Preparations & dosage: *Infusion:* Pour 1 cup of boiling water onto 1 to 2 tsp. of the dried herb and leave to infuse for 10 to 15 minutes. This should be taken as hot as possible. During fevers or the flu it should be taken every half hour. *Tincture:* Take ½ tsp. of the tincture 3 times a day.

CALIFORNIA POPPY   *Eschscholzia californica*
Part used: Dried aerial parts.
Actions: Nervine, hypnotic, antispasmodic, anodyne.
Indications: A good general relaxing herb, it has been used as a sedative and hypnotic for children, where there is overexcitability and sleeplessness. It can be used wherever an antispasmodic remedy is required.
Preparations & dosage: *Infusion:* Pour 1 cup of boiling water onto 1 to 2 tsp. of the dried herb and leave to infuse for 10 minutes. A cup should be taken at night to promote restful sleep. *Tincture:* Take ½ tsp. of the tincture at night.

CHAMOMILE   *Matricaria recutita*
Part used: Flowering tops.
Actions: Nervine, antispasmodic, carminative, anti-inflammatory, antimicrobial, bitter, vulnerary.
Indications: A comprehensive list of chamomile's medical uses would be very long. Included would be insomnia, anxiety, menopausal depression, loss of appetite, dyspep-

sia, diarrhea, colic, aches and pains of flu, migraine, neuralgia, teething, vertigo, motion sickness, conjunctivitis,
inflamed skin, urticaria and more. This may seem too good
to be true, but it reflects the wide range of actions in
the body.

Chamomile is probably the most widely used relaxing
nervine herb in the Western world. It relaxes and tones
the nervous system, and is especially valuable where anxiety and tension produce digestive symptoms such as gas,
colic pains or even ulcers. The ability to focus on physical
symptoms as well as underlying psychological tension is
one of the great benefits of herbal remedies in stress and
anxiety problems. Safe in all types of stress and anxiety-
related problems, chamomile makes a wonderful late night
tea to ensure restful sleep. It is helpful for anxious children
or teething infants, where it is used as an addition to the
bath.

As an antispasmodic herb, it works on the peripheral
nerves and muscles and so it indirectly relaxes the whole
body. When the physical body is at ease, ease in the mind
and heart follows. It can prevent or ease cramps in the
muscles, such as in the leg or abdomen. As an essential
oil added to a bath, it relaxes the body after a hard day
while easing the cares and weight of a troubled heart
and mind.

Being rich in essential oil, chamomile acts on the digestive system, promoting proper function. This usually in-
volves soothing the walls of the intestines, easing griping
pains and helping with the removal of gas. It is an effective anti-inflammatory remedy when taken internally for
the digestive and respiratory system as well as when used
externally on the skin. A cup of hot chamomile tea is a
simple, effective way to relieve indigestion, calm inflammation such as gastritis and help prevent ulcer formation.
Using the essential oil as a steam inhalation will allow the

same oils to reach inflamed mucous membranes in the sinuses and lungs.

Clinical and laboratory research demonstrates statistically what the herbalist knows experientially, that chamomile will reduce inflammation, colic pain and protect against ulcer formation in the whole of the digestive tract. **Preparations & dosage:** The herb may be used in all the ways plants can be prepared as medicines. Used fresh or dried it can be infused to make a tea. The tincture is an excellent way of ensuring that all the plant's components are extracted and available for the body. In aromatherapy the essential oil of chamomile is a valued preparation. *Tea:* Take 2 to 3 tsp. dried herb infused in 1 cup boiling water for 10 minutes, 3 to 4 times a day. *Tincture:* Take ¼ tsp. 3 times a day.

CRAMPBARK   *Viburnum opulus*
Part used: Dried bark.
Actions: Antispasmodic, anti-inflammatory, nervine, hypotensive, astringent.
Indications: Crampbark shows by its name its richly deserved reputation as a relaxer of muscular tension and spasm. It has two main areas of use, in muscular cramps and in ovarian and uterine muscle problems. Crampbark will relax the uterus and so relieve painful cramps associated with menstrual periods. In a similar way it may be used to protect from threatened miscarriage. Its astringent action gives it a role in the treatment of excessive blood loss, especially bleeding associated with the menopause.
Preparations & dosage: *Decoction:* Put 2 tsp. of the dried bark into 1 cup of water and bring to boil. Simmer gently for 10 to 15 minutes. Strain. Drink a hot cup of this tea 3 times a day. *Tincture:* Take ½ tsp. 3 times a day.

ECHINACEA   *Echinacea spp.*
Part used: Root.
Actions: Antimicrobial, immunomodulator, anticatarrhal, alterative.
Indications: Echinacea is one of the primary remedies for helping the body rid itself of microbial infections. It is often effective against both bacterial and viral attacks, and may be used in conditions such as boils, septicemia and similar infections. In conjunction with other herbs it may be used for any infection anywhere in the body. For example in combination with yarrow or bearberry it will effectively stop cystitis. It is especially useful for infections of the upper respiratory tract such as laryngitis, tonsillitis and for catarrhal conditions of the nose and sinus. In general it may be used widely and safely. The tincture or decoction may be used as a mouthwash in the treatment of pyorrhoea and gingivitis. It may also be used as an external lotion to help septic sores and cuts.
Preparations & dosage: *Decoction:* Put 1 to 2 tsp. of the root in 1 cup of water and bring it slowly to boil. Let it simmer for 10 to 15 minutes. Strain. Drink 3 times a day. *Tincture:* Take ¼ to ½ tsp. 3 times a day.

ELDER   *Sambucus nigra*
Part used: Bark, flowers, berries, leaves.
Actions: *Bark:* Purgative, emetic, diuretic. *Leaves:* Externally emollient and vulnerary, internally as purgative, expectorant, diuretic and diaphoretic. *Flowers:* Diaphoretic, anticatarrhal, antispasmodic. *Berries:* Diaphoretic, diuretic, laxative.
Indications: The elder tree is a medicine chest by itself! The leaves are used for bruises, sprains, wounds and chilblains. It has been reported that elder leaves may be useful in an ointment for tumors. Elder flowers are ideal for the treatment of colds and influenza. They are indicated in any catarrhal

inflammation of the upper respiratory tract such as hay fever and sinusitis. Catarrhal deafness responds well to elder flowers. Elderberries have similar properties to the flowers with the addition of their usefulness in rheumatism.

Combinations: For colds and fevers it may be used with peppermint, yarrow or hyssop. For influenza combine it with boneset. For catarrhal states mix it with goldenrod.

Preparations & dosage: *Infusion:* Pour 1 cup of boiling water onto 2 tsp. of the dried or fresh blossoms and infuse for 10 minutes. Drink hot 3 times a day. *Juice:* Boil fresh berries in water for 2 to 3 minutes, then express the juice. To preserve, bring to the boil with 1 part honey to 10 parts of juice. Take 1 cup diluted with hot water twice a day. *Ointment:* Take 3 parts of fresh elder leaves and heat them with 6 parts of melted Vaseline until the leaves are crisp. Strain and store. *Tincture:* Take ¼ tsp. of the tincture (made from the flowers) 3 times a day.

EYEBRIGHT *Euphrasia officinalis*
Part used: Dried aerial parts.
Actions: Anticatarrhal, astringent, anti-inflammatory.
Indications: Eyebright is an excellent remedy for the problems of mucous membranes. The combination of anti-inflammatory and astringent properties make it relevant in many conditions. Used internally it is a powerful anticatarrhal and thus may be used to treat nasal catarrh, sinusitis and other congestive states. It is best known for its use in conditions of the eye, where it is helpful in acute or chronic inflammations, stinging and weeping eyes as well as oversensitivity to light. Used as a compress externally in conjunction with internal use, it is valuable in conjunctivitis and blepharitis.
Combinations: In catarrhal conditions it combines well with goldenrod, elder flower or goldenseal. In allergic conditions where the eyes are affected it may be combined

with ephedra. As an eye lotion it may be mixed with goldenseal and distilled witch hazel.

Preparations & dosage: *Infusion:* Pour a cup of boiling water onto 1 tsp. of the dried herb and leave to infuse for 5-10 minutes. Strain. Drink 3 times a day. *Compress:* Place 1 tsp. of the dried herb in 1 pint of water and boil for 10 minutes, let cool slightly and strain. Moisten a compress (cotton wool, gauze or muslin) in the luke-warm liquid, wring out slightly and place over the eyes. Leave the compress in place for 15 minutes. Repeat several times a day. *Tincture:* Take ¼ tsp. 3 times a day.

FEVERFEW *Tanacetum parthenium*
Part used: Leaves.
Actions: Anti-inflammatory, vasodilator, bitter, emmenagogue.
Indications: Feverfew has regained its deserved reputation as a primary remedy in the treatment of migraine headaches, especially those that are relieved by applying warmth to the head. It may also help arthritis in the painfully active inflammatory stage. Dizziness and tinnitus may be eased, especially if it is used in conjunction with other remedies. Painful periods and sluggish menstrual flow will be relieved by feverfew. It is the only herb used in European phytotherapy known to be specific for the treatment of migraine. It is also the best example of a remedy well known to medical herbalists that has recently been accepted and used by allopathic medicine. It has been used throughout recorded medical history as a bitter tonic and remedy for severe headaches.
Preparation & dosage: It is best to use the equivalent of one fresh leaf 1–3 times a day. Preferably use fresh, but tincture or tablets are adequate. In this case, freeze-dried leaf preparations will be best (50–100 mg a day).

GINKGO   *Ginkgo biloba*
Part used: Leaves.
Actions: Anti-inflammatory, vasodilator.
Indications: Recent research has confirmed ginkgo's profound activity on brain function and cerebral circulation and clinically it is proving effective in a range of vascular disorders, especially those due to restricted cerebral blood flow and milder problems of normal aging such as weak memory, poor concentration and depression. Ginkgo has been suggested for a wide range of conditions: vertigo, tinnitus, inner ear disturbances including partial deafness, impairment of memory and ability to concentrate, diminished intellectual capacity and alertness as a result of insufficient circulation, dementia, Alzheimer's disease, complications of stroke and skull injuries, diminished sight and hearing ability due to vascular insufficiency, intermittent claudication as a result of arterial obstruction, Raynaud's disease and cerebral vascular and nutritional insufficiency.
Preparations & dosage: Ginkgo is becoming available in a number of different forms. The daily dose used in most studies is 27 mg of ginkgo flavone glycosides, which corresponds to 6 to 12g of leaf, depending on the quality of the leaf. Products are usually standardized to contain 24 percent flavone glycosides and hence are highly concentrated compared to the original leaf. It is recommended at a dose of 120 mg daily in two to three divided doses.

GINGER   *Zingiber officinale*
Part used: The rootstock.
Actions: Stimulant, carminative, antispasmodic, rubefacient, diaphoretic, emmenagogue.
Indications: Ginger may be used as a stimulant of the peripheral circulation in cases of circulation, chilblains and cramps. In feverish conditions, ginger acts as a useful diaphoretic, promoting perspiration. As a gargle it may be ef-

fective in the relief of sore throats. Externally it is the basis of many fibrositis and muscle sprain treatments. Ginger has been used worldwide as an aromatic carminative and pungent appetite stimulant. In India, and in other countries with hot and humid climates, ginger is eaten daily and is a well-known remedy for digestion problems. Its widespread use is not only due to its lively flavor, but to its antioxidant and antimicrobial effects, necessary for the preservation of food, which is essential in such climates.

Preparations & dosage: *Infusion:* Pour 1 cup of boiling water onto 1 tsp. of the fresh root and let it infuse for 5 minutes. Drink whenever needed. *Decoction:* If you are using the dried root in powdered or finely chopped form, make a decoction by putting 1½ tsp in 1 cup of water. Bring it to the boil and simmer for 5 to 10 minutes. Drink whenever needed.

GINSENG, Korean and American   *Panax spp.*
Part used: Root.
Actions: Adaptogen, tonic, stimulant, hypoglycemic.
Indications: Ginseng has an ancient history and as such has accumulated much folklore about its actions and uses. The genus name *panax* derives from the Latin *panacea* meaning "cure all." Many of the claims that surround it are, unfortunately, exaggerated, but it is clear that this is an important remedy. A powerful adaptogen, it has a wide range of possible therapeutic uses. The best therapeutic application is with weak or elderly people, where the adaptogenic and stimulating properties can be profoundly useful. It should not be used indiscriminately as the stimulating properties can be contraindicated in some pathologies; for example, Chinese herbalism warns about ginseng being used in acute inflammatory disease and bronchitis.

Preparations & dosage: *Decoction:* Put ½ to 1 tsp. of the root in 1 cup of water, bring to the boil and simmer gently for 10 minutes. Strain and drink 3 times a day. *Tincture:* Take ¼ tsp. 3 times a day for up to 3 months.

GOLDENROD   *Solidago virgaurea*
Part used: Dried aerial parts.
Actions: Anticatarrhal, anti-inflammatory, antimicrobial, astringent, diaphoretic, carminative, diuretic.
Indications: Goldenrod is perhaps the first plant to think of for upper respiratory catarrh, whether acute or chronic; it may be used in combination with other herbs in the treatment of influenza. The carminative properties reveal a role in the treatment of flatulent dyspepsia. As an anti-inflammatory urinary antiseptic, Goldenrod may be used in cystitis, urethritis and the like. It can be used to promote the healing of wounds. As a gargle it can be used in laryngitis and pharyngitis.
Combinations: For upper respiratory catarrh it may be used with eyebright, elder, echinacea, poke root and wild indigo.
Preparations & dosage: *Infusion:* Pour 1 cup of boiling water onto 2 to 3 tsp. of the dried herb and leave to infuse for 10 to 15 minutes. Strain and drink 3 times a day. *Tincture:* Take ½ tsp. 3 times a day.

HOPS   *Humulus lupulus*
Part used: Flower inflorescence.
Actions: Sedative, hypnotic, antimicrobial, antispasmodic, astringent.
Indications: Hops is a remedy that has a marked relaxing effect upon the central nervous system. It is used extensively for the treatment of insomnia. It will ease tension and anxiety and may be used where tension leads to restlessness, headache and possibly indigestion. As an astringent with these relaxing properties it can be used in conditions such as mucous colitis. It should, however, be avoided where there is a marked degree of depression as

this may be accentuated. Externally, the antiseptic action of hops is utilized for the treatment of ulcers.

CAUTION: Do not use in cases of depression.

Preparations & dosage: *Infusion:* Pour 1 cup of boiling water onto 1 tsp. of the dried flowers and let infuse for 10 to 15 minutes. Drink at night to induce sleep. This dose may be strengthened if needed. *Tincture:* Take ¼ tsp. 3 times a day.

HYSSOP   *Hyssopus officinalis*
Part used: Dried aerial parts.
Actions: Antispasmodic, expectorant, diaphoretic, nervine, anti-inflammatory, carminative.
Indications: Hyssop has an interesting range of uses which are largely attributable to the antispasmodic action of the volatile oil. It is used in coughs, bronchitis and chronic catarrh. Its diaphoretic properties explain its use in the common cold. As a nervine it may be used in anxiety states, hysteria and petit mal (a form of epilepsy).
Preparations & dosage: *Infusion:* Pour a cup of boiling water onto 1 to 2 tsp. of the dried herb and leave to infuse for 10 to 15 minutes. Strain and drink 3 times a day. *Tincture:* Take ¼ tsp. 3 times a day.

KAVA KAVA   *Piper methysticum*
Part used: Rhizome.
Actions: Relaxing nervine, hypnotic, antispasmodic, local anesthetic, antifungal.
Indications: Kava kava is a safe treatment for anxiety. At normal therapeutic doses it does not dampen alertness or interact with mild alcohol consumption. It possesses a mild antidepressant activity, making it suitable for the treatment of anxiety associated with minor forms of depression. Kava is an effective muscle relaxant, making it useful for the treatment of conditions associated with skeletal muscle

spasm and tension, such as headaches due to neck tension. It is also a relevant hypnotic in cases of mild insomnia. The local anesthetic action on mucous membranes makes kava useful for pain control in oral conditions.

Preparations & dosage: *Decoction.* Put 1 to 2 tsp. of the rhizome in 1 cup of water, bring to boil and simmer gently for 10 to 15 minutes; drink as needed. *Tincture:* Take ½ tsp. per day. Standardized preparations should supply 100 to 200 mg of kava lactones per day.

KOLA   *Cola vera*
Part used: Seed kernel.

Actions: Stimulant to central nervous system, antidepressive, astringent, diuretic.

Indications: Kola has a marked stimulating effect on human consciousness. It can be used wherever there is a need for direct stimulation, which is less often than is usually thought, since, with good health and therefore right functioning, the nervous system does not need such help. In the short term it may be used in nervous debility, in states of atony and weakness. It can act as a specific in nervous diarrhea. It will aid in states of depression and may, in some people, give rise to euphoric states. In some varieties of migraine it can help greatly. It can be viewed as a specific in cases of depression associated with weakness and debility.

Preparations & dosage: *Decoction:* Put 1 to 2 tsp. of the powdered nuts in a cup of water, bring to boil and simmer gently for 10 to 15 minutes. Drink when needed. *Tincture:* Take ¼ to ½ tsp. of the tincture 3 times a day.

LAVENDER   *Lavandula officinalis*
Part used: Flowers.

Actions: Carminative, antispasmodic, antidepressant, emmenagogue, hypotensive.

Indications: This beautiful herb has many uses, culinary, cosmetic and medicinal. It is often an effective herb for headaches, especially when they are related to stress. Lavender can be quite effective in the clearing of depression, especially if used in conjunction with other remedies. As a gentle strengthening tonic of the nervous system it may be used in states of nervous debility and exhaustion. It can be used to soothe and promote natural sleep. Externally the oil may be used as a stimulating liniment to help ease the aches and pains of rheumatism.

Preparations & dosage: *Infusion:* To take internally, pour 1 cup of boiling water onto 1 tsp. of the dried herb and leave to infuse for 10 minutes. Strain and drink 3 times a day. *External use:* The oil should not be taken internally but can be inhaled, rubbed on the skin or used in baths.

LEMON BALM   *Melissa officinalis*
Part used: Dried aerial parts, or fresh in season.
Actions: Carminative, nervine, antispasmodic, diaphoretic, antimicrobial.
Indications: Lemon balm is a relaxing, carminative herb that relieves spasms in the digestive tract and is often used in flatulent dyspepsia. It is especially helpful where there is dyspepsia associated with anxiety or depression, as the gently sedative oils relieve tension and anxiety reactions. It may also be used in migraine that is associated with tension, neuralgia, anxiety-induced palpitations and insomnia. Extracts have antiviral properties, and a lotion based extract may be used for the skin lesions of herpes simplex, the antiviral activity having been confirmed in both laboratory and clinical trials.

Preparations & dosage: *Infusion:* Pour 1 cup of boiling water onto 1 to 2 tsp. of the dried herb or 4 to 6 fresh leaves and leave to infuse for 10 to 15 minutes, well-covered. A cup of this tea should be taken in the morning and the evening, or when needed. *Tincture:* Take ¼ tsp. 3 times a day.

LINDEN   *Tilia europea*
Part used: Dried flowers.
Actions: Nervine, antispasmodic, hypotensive, diaphoretic, diuretic, anti-inflammatory, astringent.
Indications: Linden is well known as a relaxing remedy for use in nervous tension. It has a reputation as a prophylactic against the development of arteriosclerosis and hypertension. It is considered a specific in the treatment of raised blood pressure associated with arteriosclerosis and nervous tension. Its relaxing action, combined with a general effect upon the circulatory system give linden a role in the treatment of some forms of migraine. Linden's diaphoretic action combined with its relaxing effects explain its value in feverish colds and flu.
Preparations & dosage: *Infusion:* Pour 1 cup of boiling water onto 1 tsp. of the blossoms and leave to infuse for 10 minutes. Strain and drink 3 times a day. For a diaphoretic effect in fever, use 2 to 3 tsp. *Tincture:* Take ¼ tsp. 3 times a day.

MEADOWSWEET   *Filipendula ulmaria*
Part used: Aerial parts.
Actions: Antirheumatic, anti-inflammatory, carminative, antacid, antiemetic, astringent.
Indications: Meadowsweet is one of the best digestive remedies available and as such is indicated in many conditions if they are approached holistically. It acts to protect and soothe the mucous membranes of the digestive tract, reducing excess acidity and easing nausea. It is used in the treatment of heartburn, hyperacidity, gastritis and peptic ulceration. Its gentle astringency is useful in treating diarrhea in children. The presence of aspirin-like chemicals

explains meadowsweet's action in reducing fever and relieving the pain of rheumatism in muscles and joints.

Combinations: With marshmallow and chamomile it is very soothing for a whole range of digestive problems. For musculoskeletal conditions consider combining with black cohosh, willow bark and celery seed for its anti-inflammatory effects.

Preparations & dosage: *Infusion:* Pour 1 cup of boiling water onto 1 to 2 tsp. of the dried herb and leave to infuse for 10 to 15 minutes. Strain and drink 3 times a day or as needed. *Tincture:* Take ¼ to ½ tsp. 3 times a day.

MUGWORT   *Artemisia vulgaris*
Part used: Leaves or root.

Actions: Bitter tonic, nervine tonic, emmenagogue.

Indications: Mugwort can be used wherever a digestive stimulant is called for. It will aid digestion through the bitter stimulation of its juices while its oils provide a carminative effect. It has a mildly nervine action in aiding depression and easing tension which appears to be due to the volatile oil, so it is essential that this not be lost in preparation. Mugwort may also be used as an emmenagogue to aid normal menstrual flow.

Preparations & dosage: *Infusion:* Pour 1 cup of boiling water onto 1 to 2 tsp. of the dried herb and leave to infuse for 10 to 15 minutes in a covered container. Strain and drink 3 times a day. Mugwort is used as flavoring in a number of aperitif drinks such as vermouth, a pleasant way to take it. *Tincture:* ¼ tsp. 3 times a day.

OATS   *Avena sativa*
Part used: Seeds and whole plant.

Actions: Nervine tonic, antidepressant, nutritive, demulcent, vulnerary.

Indications: Oats is one of the best remedies for "feeding" the nervous system, especially when under stress. It is considered a specific in cases of nervous debility and exhaustion when associated with depression. It may be used with most of the other nervines, both relaxant and stimulatory, to strengthen the whole of the nervous system. It is also used in general debility.

Preparations & dosage: *Infusion:* Pour a cup of boiling water onto 1 to 3 tsp. of the dried oatstraw and leave to infuse 10 to 15 minutes. Strain and drink 3 times a day. *Tincture:* Take ½ tsp. 3 times a day. *Bath:* A soothing bath for use in neuralgia and irritated skin conditions can be made. Boil 1 pound of shredded oatstraw in 2 quarts of water for half an hour. Strain and add to the bath. Alternatively, cooked rolled oats may be put into a muslin bag and used to bathe with.

PULSATILLA   *Anemone pulsatilla*
Part used: Aerial parts.
Actions: Nervine, antispasmodic, antibacterial.
Indications: Pulsatilla is an excellent relaxing nervine for use in problems related to nervous tension and spasm in the reproductive system. It may be used with safety in the relief of painful periods (dysmenorrhea), ovarian pain and painful conditions of the testes. It may be used to reduce tension and headaches associated with tension. It will help ease insomnia and general hyperactivity. Its antibacterial action gives this herb a role in treating infections that affect the skin, especially boils. It is similarly useful in the treatment of respiratory infections and asthma. The oil or tincture will ease earache.

Preparations & dosage: *Infusion:* Pour 1 cup of boiling water onto ½ to 1 tsp. of the dried herb and leave to infuse for 10 to 15 minutes. Strain and drink 3 times a day or when needed. *Tincture:* Take ¼ tsp. 3 times a day.

PASSIONFLOWER   *Passiflora incarnata*
Part used: Leaves and whole plant.

Actions: Nervine, hypnotic, antispasmodic, anodyne, hypotensive.

Indications: Passionflower has a depressant effect on central nervous system activity, is hypotensive and is used for its sedative and soothing properties to lower blood pressure and ease insomnia. The alkaloids and flavonoids have both been reported to have sedative activity in animals. Many of the flavonoids, such as *apigenin,* are well known for pharmacological activity, particularly antispasmodic and anti-inflammatory activities. It is the herb of choice for treating intransigent insomnia. It aids the transition into a restful sleep without any narcotic hangover. It may be used wherever an antispasmodic is required, e.g., in Parkinson's disease, seizures and hysteria. It can help to relieve nerve pain such as neuralgia and shingles, a viral infection of the nerves.

Preparations & dosage: *Infusion:* Pour 1 cup of boiling water onto 1 to 2 tsp. of the dried herb and let infuse for 15 minutes. Drink a cup in the evening for sleeplessness and a cup twice a day for the easing of other conditions. *Tincture:* Take ¼ tsp. and use the same way as the infusion.

PEPPERMINT   *Mentha piperita*
Part used: Aerial parts.

Actions: Carminative, anti-inflammatory, antispasmodic, aromatic, diaphoretic, antiemetic, nervine, antimicrobial, analgesic.

Indications: Peppermint is an excellent carminative, with a relaxing effect on the muscles of the digestive system; it combats flatulence and stimulates bile and digestive juice flow. It is used to relieve intestinal colic, flatulent dyspepsia and associated conditions. The volatile oil acts as a mild anesthetic to the stomach wall, which allays feelings of nausea and the urge to vomit. It helps to relieve the nausea and vomiting of pregnancy and travel sickness. Peppermint can play a role in the treatment of ulcerative conditions of the bowels. It is a traditional treatment for fevers, colds and influenza. As an inhalant it is used as temporary relief for nasal catarrh. Where headaches are associated with digestion, peppermint may help. As a nervine it eases anxiety and tension. In painful periods, it relieves the pain and eases associated tension. Externally it is used to relieve itching and inflammation.

Preparations & dosage: *Infusion:* Pour 1 cup of boiling water onto a heaped teaspoonful of the dried herb and leave to infuse for 10 minutes. Strain and drink as often as desired. *Tincture:* Take ¼ tsp. 3 times a day.

PRICKLY ASH   *Zanthoxylum americanum*
Part used: The bark and berries.
Actions: Stimulant (circulatory), tonic, alterative, carminative, diaphoretic, antirheumatic, hepatic.
Indications: Prickly ash may be used in a way that is similar to cayenne, although it is slower in action. It is used in many chronic problems such as rheumatism and skin diseases. Any sign of poor circulation calls for the use of this herb, such as chilblains, leg cramps, varicose veins and varicose ulcers. Externally it may be used as a stimulating liniment for rheumatism and fibrositis. Due to its stimulating effect on the lymphatic system, circulation and mucous membranes, it has a role in the holistic treatment of many specific conditions.
Preparations & dosage: *Infusion:* Pour 1 cup of boiling water onto 1 to 2 tsp. of the bark and let infuse for 10 to 15 minutes. Strain and drink 3 times a day. *Tincture:* Take ¼ to ½ tsp. 3 times a day.

SIBERIAN GINSENG   *Eleutherococcus senticosus*
Part used: The root.
Actions: Adaptogen.
Indications: Siberian ginseng can be recommended as a

general tonic for a very wide range of clinical indications because of its nonspecific action. It is especially useful in conditions impacted by the stress response, including angina, hypertension, hypotension, various types of neuroses, chronic bronchitis and cancer. Siberian ginseng is also used to treat the effects of prolonged stress or overwork such as exhaustion, irritability, insomnia and mild depression. It can be used to assist recovery from acute or chronic diseases, trauma, surgery and other stressful episodes as well as to counter the debilitating effects of chronic disease and treatments such as chemotherapy and radiation. It can be taken on a long-term basis to minimize the incidence of acute infections and to generally improve well-being.

Preparations & dosage: *Tincture:* The standard dosage, based upon clinical studies, is ½ tsp. 3 times a day. *Tablet:* An equivalent dosage using a solid extract concentrated at a ratio of 20:1 would be 100 to 200 mg. The recommended regime is usually for a six-week course followed by a two-week break. This regime can be repeated for as long as is necessary.

SKULLCAP   *Scutellaria laterifolia*
Part used: Aerial parts
Actions: Nervine tonic, anti-spasmodic, hypotensive.
Indications: Skullcap is perhaps the most widely relevant nervine available to us in the materia medica. It relaxes states of nervous tension while at the same time renewing and revivifying the central nervous system. It has a specific use in the treatment of seizure and hysterical states as well as epilepsy. It may be used in all exhausted or depressed conditions. It can be used with complete safety in the easing of premenstrual tension.

Preparations & dosage: *Infusion:* Pour 1 cup boiling water onto 1 to 2 tsp. of the dried herb and leave to infuse for 10 to 15 minutes. Strain and drink 3 times a day or when needed. *Tincture:* Take ½ tsp. 3 times a day.

ST. JOHN'S WORT   *Hypericum perforatum*

Part used: Aerial parts.

Actions: Anti-inflammatory, antidepressant, astringent, vulnerary, nervine, antimicrobial.

Indications: Taken internally, St. John's wort has a sedative and mild pain-reducing effect, which gives it a place in the treatment of neuralgia, anxiety, tension and similar problems. It is especially regarded as an herb to use where there are menopausal changes triggering irritability and anxiety. It is increasingly recommended in the treatment of depression. The standardized extract is recognized as an effective treatment for depressive states, fear and nervous disturbances by the German government. In addition to neuralgic pain, it will ease fibrositis, sciatica and rheumatic pain. Externally it is a valuable healing and anti-inflammatory remedy. As a lotion it will speed the healing of wounds and bruises, varicose veins and mild burns. The oil is especially useful for the healing of sunburn.

Preparations & dosage: *Infusion:* Pour 1 cup of boiling water onto 1 to 2 tsp. of the dried herb and leave to infuse for 10 to 15 minutes. Strain and drink 3 times a day. *Tincture:* Take ¼ to ½ tsp. 3 times a day. *Tablet:* In the treatment of depression the recommended dose is 300 mg of concentrated dry extract standardized to 0.3 percent hypericin 3 times daily.

THYME   *Thymus vulgaris*

Part used: Leaves and flowering tops.

Actions: Carminative, antimicrobial, antispasmodic, expectorant, astringent, anthelmintic.

Indications: With its high content of volatile oil, thyme makes a good carminative for use in dyspepsia and sluggish digestion. This oil is also a strongly antiseptic substance, which explains many of its uses. It can be used externally as a lotion for infected wounds, but also internally for respiratory and digestive infections. It may be use as a gargle in laryngitis and tonsillitis, easing sore throats and soothing irritable coughs. It is an excellent cough remedy, producing expectoration and reducing unnecessary spasm. It may be used in bronchitis, whooping cough and asthma. A warm infusion is beneficial in headache and to promote perspiration.

Preparations & dosage: *Infusion:* Pour 1 cup of boiling water onto 2 tsp. of the dried herb and let infuse for 10 minutes. Strain and drink 3 times a day. *Tincture:* Take ½ tsp. 3 times a day.

VITEX (CHASTEBERRY)   *Vitex agnus-castus*
Part used: The fruit.
Actions: Hormonal normalizer.
Indications: Vitex or chasteberry has the effect of stimulating and normalizing pituitary gland functions, especially the progesterone function. It may be called an amphoteric remedy, as it can produce apparently opposite effects, though in truth it is simply normalizing. It has, for instance, a reputation as both an aphrodisiac and an anaphrodisiac! It will usually enable what is appropriate to occur. The greatest use of vitex lies in normalizing the activity of female sex hormones and it is thus indicated for dysmenorrhea, premenstrual stress and other disorders related to hormone function. It is especially beneficial during menopausal changes. In a similar way it may be used to aid the body to regain a natural balance after the use of the birth control pill.

Preparations & dosage: *Infusion:* Pour 1 cup of boiling water onto 1 tsp. of the ripe berries and leave to infuse for 10 to 15 minutes. Strain and drink 3 times a day. *Tincture:* Take ¼ tsp. 3 times a day.

WHITE POPLAR   *Populus tremuloides*
Part used: The bark.

Action: Anti-inflammatory, astringent, antiseptic, anodyne, cholagogue, bitter tonic.

Indications: White poplar is an excellent remedy to use in the treatment of arthritis and rheumatism where there is much pain and swelling. In this area, its use is quite similar to willow. It is most effective when used as part of a broad therapeutic approach and not by itself. It is very helpful during a flare-up of rheumatoid arthritis. As a cholagogue it can be used to stimulate digestion, especially stomach and liver function where there is loss of appetite. In feverish colds and in infections such as cystitis it may be considered. As an astringent it can be used in the treatment of diarrhea.

Preparations & dosage: *Decoction:* Put 1 to 2 tsp. of the dried bark in a cup of water, bring to the boil and simmer for 10 to 15 minutes. Strain and drink 3 times a day. To stimulate appetite, drink 30 minutes before meals.*Tincture:* Take ½ tsp. 3 times a day.

WILD CHERRY BARK   *Prunus serotina*
Part used: Dried bark.

Actions: Antitussive, expectorant, astringent, nervine, antispasmodic.

Indications: While this herb is not a directly relaxing remedy, it may be used for easing stress or tension induced by coughing or asthma. Due to its powerful sedative action on the cough reflex, wild cherry bark finds its main use in the treatment of irritating coughs and thus has a role in the treatment of bronchitis and whooping cough. It can be used with other herbs in the control of asthma. It must be remembered, however, that the inhibition of a cough does not equate with the healing of a chest infection, which will still need to be treated. It may also be used as a bitter when digestion is sluggish. The cold infusion of the bark may be helpful as a wash in cases of eye inflammation.

Preparations & dosage: *Infusion:* Pour 1 cup of boiling water onto 1 to 2 tsp. of the dried bark and leave to infuse for 10 to 15 minutes. Strain and drink 3 times a day. *Tinctures:* Take ¼ tsp. 3 times a day.

WILD INDIGO   *Baptisia tinctoria*
Part used: Root.

Actions: Antimicrobial, anticatarrhal.

Indications: Wild indigo is an herb to be considered wherever there is a focused infection. It is especially useful in the treatment of infections and catarrh in the ear, nose and throat. It may be used for laryngitis, tonsillitis, pharyngitis and catarrhal infections of the nose and sinuses. Taken both internally and as a mouthwash it will heal mouth ulcers and gingivitis and help in the control of pyorrhea. Systemically it may be helpful to treat enlarged and inflamed lymph glands and also to reduce fevers. Externally an ointment will help infected ulcers and ease sore nipples. A douche of the concoction will help leucorrhea.

Preparations & dosage: *Decoction:* Put ½ to 1 tsp. of the dried root in 1 cup of water, bring to the boil and simmer for 10 to 15 minutes. Strain and drink 3 times a day. *Tincture:* Take ¼ tsp. 3 times a day.

WILD LETTUCE   *Lactuca virosa*
Part used: Dried leaves.

Actions: Nervine, anodyne, hypnotic, antispasmodic.

Indications: The latex of the wild lettuce was at one time sold as "Lettuce Opium," naming the use of this herb quite well! It is a valuable remedy for use in insomnia, restlessness and excitability (especially in children) and other manifestations of an overactive nervous system. As an antispasmodic it can be used as part of a holistic treatment of whooping cough and dry irritated coughs in general. It will relieve colic pains in the intestines and uterus and so may be used in dysmenorrhea. It will ease muscular pains related to rheumatism. It has been used as an anaphrodisiac.

Combinations: For irritable coughs it may be used with wild cherry bark. For insomnia it combines with valerian and pulsatilla.

Preparations & dosage: *Infusion:* Pour 1 cup of boiling water onto 1 to 2 tsp. of the leaves and let infuse for 10 to 15 minutes. Strain and drink 3 times a day. *Tincture:* Take ¼ to ½ tsp. 3 times a day.

WILLOW   *Salix spp.*
Part used: Bark
Actions: Analgesic, anti-inflammatory, antipyretic, astringent, tonic.
Indications: Willow is an ancient remedy which has been used in various forms for rheumatism, gout, fevers and aches and pains of all kinds. It is often considered to be the natural form of aspirin. However, as described elsewhere, this is not strictly true. It can be taken internally for arthritic complaints and gout, headaches, fever due to common colds or influenza, and as an aid in treating mild diarrhea, general neuralgia and hay fever. Applied externally, a poultice or fomentation can be used to ease the pain of arthritic joints and as a wash for sores and burns.
Preparations & dosage: *Infusion:* Pour 1 cup of boiling water onto 1 to 2 tsp. of the dried herb and leave to infuse for 10 to 15 minutes. Strain and drink 3 times a day. *Tincture:* Take ½ tsp. 3 times a day.

WOOD BETONY   *Betonica officinalis*
Part used: Dried aerial parts.
Actions: Nervine, bitter.

Indication: Betony gently tones and strengthens the nervous system and also has a relaxing action if used in nervous debility associated with anxiety and tension. It will ease headaches and neuralgia when they are of nervous origin, especially when caused by hypertension.

Combinations: For the treatment of nervous headaches it combines well with skullcap. In hypertensive headaches use in combination with appropriate hypotensives.

Preparations & dosage: *Infusion:* Pour 1 cup of boiling water onto 1 to 2 tsp. of the dried herb and leave to infuse for 10 to 15 minutes. Strain and drink 3 times a day. *Tincture:* Take ½ tsp. 3 times a day.

The Preparation of Herbal Medicines

From a therapeutic perspective, the basic way to use herbs is to take them internally since it is from within that healing takes place. The ways to prepare internal remedies are numerous, but with all of them it is essential to prepare carefully to ensure you end up with a medicine that works.

TEAS

There are two ways to prepare teas: as infusions or decoctions. There are some basic rules of thumb for choosing which method to use with what herb, but as with all generalizations, there are many exceptions.

Infusions are usually appropriate for non-woody material such as leaves, flowers and some stems.

Decoctions are usually required if the herb contains any hard or woody material such as roots, barks or nuts. The denser the plant or the individual cell walls, the more energy is needed to extract cell content into the tea, thus explaining the value of decocting. An important exception would be a root rich in a volatile oil such as valerian. The woodiness of valerian root would suggest decocting, but if the roots were simmered the therapeutically important volatile oil would boil off.

To Make an Infusion

- Take a china or glass teapot which has been warmed and put about one teaspoonful of the dried herb or herb mixture into it for each cup of tea.
- Pour a cup of boiling water in the pot for each teaspoonful of herb and then put the lid on. Steep for 10 to 15 minutes. Infusions may be taken hot which is normally best for a medicinal herb tea, cold or even iced. They may be sweetened with licorice root, honey or brown sugar. Any aromatic herb should be infused in a pot that has a tightly fitting lid to ensure that only a minimum of volatile oil is lost through evaporation.

Herbal tea bags can be made by filling little muslin bags with herbal mixtures, taking care to remember how many teaspoonsful have been put into each bag. They can be used in the same way as ordinary tea bags.

To Make a Decoction

- Put one teaspoonful of dried herb or three teaspoons of fresh material into a pot or saucepan for each cup of water. Dried herbs should be powdered or broken into small pieces, while fresh material should be cut into small pieces. If large quantities are made, use one ounce of dried herb for each pint of water. The container should be glass, ceramic or earthenware. If using metal, it should be enameled.
- Add the appropriate amount of water to the herbs.
- Bring to a boil and simmer for the time given for the mixture or specific herb, usually 10 to 15 minutes. If

the herb contains volatile oils, cover the pot with a tight-fitting lid.
- Strain the tea while still hot.

TINCTURES

In general, alcohol is a better solvent than water for plant constituents. Mixtures of alcohol and water dissolve nearly all the relevant ingredients of an herb and at the same time the alcohol acts as a preservative. Alcohol preparations are called tinctures, a word that is occasionally also used for preparations with a glycerin or vinegar base, as described below. The method given below for the preparation of tinctures shows a simple and general approach; when tinctures are prepared professionally according to descriptions in a pharmacopoeia, specific water/alcohol proportions are used for each herb, but for general use such details are unnecessary. For home use it is best to take an alcohol of at least 30 percent (60 proof), vodka for instance, as this is about the weakest alcohol/water mixture with a long-term preservative action.

To Make an Alcohol-based Tincture:

- Put 4 ounces of finely chopped or ground dried herb into a container that can be tightly closed. If fresh herbs are used, twice the amount should be used.
- Pour 1 pint of 30 percent (60 proof) vodka on the herbs and close tightly.
- Keep the container in a warm place for two weeks and shake it well twice every day.
- After decanting the bulk of the liquid, pour the residue into a muslin cloth suspended in a bowl.

- Wring out all the liquid. The residue makes excellent compost.
- Pour the tincture into a dark bottle. It should be kept well-stoppered.

As tinctures are stronger than infusions or decoctions, the dosage to be taken is much smaller, depending on the herb. Tinctures may be used in a variety of ways. They can be taken straight, mixed with water, or they can be added to a cup of hot water. If this is done, the alcohol will largely evaporate, leaving most of the extract in the water and possibly making the water cloudy, as resins and other constituents not soluble in water will precipitate. Some drops of the tincture may be added to a bath or footbath, used in a compress or mixed with oil and fat to make an ointment.

Another form of alcohol-based medicine is the liquid extract, also known as a fluid extract. It is much more concentrated than tinctures with one part by volume of the fluid extract being equivalent to one part by weight of the herb.

Another way of making an alcohol-based preparation is to infuse herbs in wine. Even though wine-based preparations do not have the shelf life of tinctures and are not as concentrated, they can be both pleasant to take and effective.

To Make a Glycerin-based Tincture

Tinctures based on glycerin have the advantage of being milder on the digestive tract and do not involve the problems associated with alcohol abuse. However, they have the disadvantage of not dissolving resinous or oily materials as well. As a solvent, glycerin is generally better than water but not as good as alcohol.

To make a glycerin tincture, make up 1 pint of a mixture consisting of one part glycerin and one part water; add 4 ounces of the dried ground herb and leave it in a well-stoppered container for two weeks, shaking it daily. After two weeks, strain and press or wring the residue as with alcoholic tinctures. For fresh herbs, due to their greater water content, put 8 oz. into a mixture of 75 percent glycerin/25 percent water.

DRY PREPARATIONS

Sometimes it is more appropriate to take herbs in a dry form, such as in capsules or tablets. There may be an advantage to this as the taste of the herb can be avoided, and the whole herb may be taken, including the woody material. There are, however, a number of drawbacks.

Because dry herbs are unprocessed, the plant constituents might not be readily available for easy absorption. During infusion, heat and water help to break down the walls of the plant cells and dissolve the constituents, a process that is not always guaranteed during the digestion process in the stomach and small intestine. When the constituents are already dissolved in liquid form, they are available a lot faster and begin their action sooner.

Taking all this into account, there are still a number of ways to use herbs in dry form. The main thing is to ensure that the herbs are powdered as finely as possible. This guarantees that the cell walls are largely broken down and aids digestion and absorption of the herb. Techniques used to grind the herb fine enough will also cause much heat generation through friction, which may lead to a change in chemistry. This change is usually an inappropriate one.

Capsules

The easiest way to take dry powdered herbs internally is to use gelatin capsules. Capsules not made of animal products are also available. The size needed depends on the amount of herbs prescribed per dose, the density of the plant and the volume of the material. A capsule size 00 holds about 0.5 grams (⅙ ounce) of finely powdered herb.

- Place the powdered herbs in a flat dish and take the halves of the capsule apart.
- Move the halves of the capsules through the powder, filling them in the process.
- Push the halves together.

Pills

There are a number of ways to make pills, depending on the degree of technical skill you possess. The simplest way to take an unpleasant-tasting remedy is to roll the powder into a small pill with fresh bread, which works most effectively with herbs such as goldenseal or cayenne.

- Grind herbs as fine as possible (a coffee grinder works well).
- Add a small amount of water and maple syrup to make a mud pie consistency.
- Knead in slippery elm powder a bit of bread to roll into small balls.

BATHS

A pleasant way to absorb herbal compounds through the skin is to take a full body bath with one pint of an infusion or decoction added to the water. Any herb that can be taken internally can also be used in a bath. Herbs can, of course, also be used to give the bath an excellent fragrance.

Appendix: Actions of Herbs

Adaptogen. An herb that increases resistance and resilience to stress, enabling the body to avoid reaching collapse because it can adapt around the problem. Adaptogens appear to work by supporting the adrenal glands.

Alterative. An herb that gradually restores proper functioning of the body, increasing health and vitality. Some alteratives support natural waste elimination via the kidneys, liver, lungs or skin. Others stimulate digestive function or are antimicrobial.

Anticatarrhal. Anticatarrhals help the body remove excess mucus, whether in the sinuses or other parts of the body. Catarrh is not of itself a problem, but when too much is produced it is usually in response to an infection or as a way for the body to remove excess carbohydrate.

Anti-inflammatory. An herb that soothes inflammations or reduces the inflammation of the tissue directly. Anti-inflammatories work in a number of different ways, but rarely inhibit the natural inflammatory reaction as such; rather they support and encourage the work the body is undertaking.

Antimicrobial. Antimicrobials help the body destroy or resist pathogenic microorganisms. Antimicrobials help the body strengthen its own resistance to infective organisms and throw off illness. While some contain either chemicals which are antiseptic or specific poisons to certain organisms, in general they aid the body's natural immunity.

Antispasmodic. Antispasmodics ease cramps in muscles. They alleviate muscular tension and, as many are also nervines, ease psychological tension as well. Some antispasmodics reduce muscle spasms throughout the body and others work on specific organs or systems.

Astringent. Astringents have a binding action on mucous membranes, skin and other tissue. The action is due to chemicals called tannins, named after their use in the tanning industry. They have the effect of precipitating protein molecules, thus reducing irritation and inflammation and creating a barrier against infection that is helpful in wounds and burns.

Bitter. Herbs with a bitter taste have a special role in preventive medicine. The taste triggers a sensory response in the central nervous system. A message goes to the gut releasing digestive hormones leading to a range of actions including stimulation of appetite, a general stimulation of the flow of digestive juices and support of the liver's detoxification work and secretion of bile flow. They also stimulate gut self-repair mechanisms.

Cardiac remedies. This is a general term for herbal remedies that have a beneficial action on the heart. Some of the remedies in this group are powerful cardioactive agents such as foxglove, whereas others are gentler, safer herbs such as hawthorn and motherwort.

Carminative. Carminatives are plants that are rich in aromatic volatile oils. They stimulate the digestive system to work properly and with ease, soothing the gut wall, reducing any inflammation that might be present, easing griping pains and helping the removal of gas from the digestive tract.

Demulcent. These are herbs rich in mucilage that soothes and protects irritated or inflamed tissue. They reduce irritation down the whole length of the bowel, reduce sensitivity to potentially corrosive gastric acids, help to prevent diarrhea and reduce the muscle spasms which cause colic. They also ease coughing by soothing bronchial tension and relax painful spasm in the bladder.

Diaphoretic. These herbs promote perspiration, helping the skin eliminate waste from the body and thus ensuring that the body has a clean and harmonious inner environment. Some produce observable sweat, while others aid normal background perspiration. They often promote dilation of surface capillaries, helping to improve poor circulation. They support the work of the kidney by increasing cleaning through the skin.

Diuretic. Diuretics increase the production and elimination of urine. In herbal medicine, with its ancient traditions, the term is often applied to herbs that have a beneficial action on the urinary system. They help the body eliminate waste and support the whole process of inner cleansing.

Emmenagogue. Emmenagogues stimulate menstrual flow and activity. In most herbals, however, the term is used in the wider sense of a remedy that normalizes and tones the female reproductive system.

Expectorant. Strictly speaking these are herbs that stimulate removal of mucus from the lungs, but the term often means a tonic for the respiratory system. Stimulating expectorants irritate the bronchioles, causing expulsion of material. Relaxing expectorants soothe bronchial spasm and loosen mucus secretions, helping in dry, irritating coughs.

Hepatic. Hepatics aid the liver. They tone, strengthen and in some cases increase the flow of bile. In a broad holistic approach to health they are of great importance because of the fundamental role of the liver in the healthy functioning of the body.

Hypotensive. These plant remedies lower abnormally elevated blood pressure.

Laxative. Laxatives stimulate bowel movements. Stimulating laxatives should not be used long term. If prolonged stimulation of the bowels appears to be necessary, then diet, general health and stress should all be closely considered.

Nervine. Nervines help the nervous system and can be meaningfully subdivided into three groups. Nervine tonics strengthen and restore the nervous system. Nervine relaxants ease anxiety and tension by soothing both body and mind. Nervine stimulants directly stimulate nerve activity.

Rubefacient. These herbs generate a localized increase in blood flow when applied to the skin, helping healing, cleansing and nourishment. They are often used to ease the pain and swelling of arthritic joints.

Tonic. Tonics nurture and enliven. Truly gifts of nature to a suffering humanity these are whole plants that enliven whole human bodies, gifts of the Mother Earth to her children. To ask how they work is to ask how life works!

Vulnerary. Vulneraries are remedies that promote wound healing. Used mainly for skin lesions, their action is just as relevant for internal wounds such as stomach ulcers.

References

1. Cutler, Robert W.P. (1993) Headache. *Sci Am.* February.
2. Stewart, et al. (1992) Prevalence of migraine headache in the United States. Relation to age, income, race, and other sociodemographic factors. *JAMA* 267:64-9.
3. Rasmussen, B.K., Olesen, J. (1992) Symptomatic and nonsymptomatic headaches in a general population. *Neurology* 42:1225.
4. Chung, M.K., Kraybill, D.E. (1990) Headache: a marker of depression. *J Fam Pract* 31:360-4.
5. Keville, K. and Green, M. *Aromatherapy. A Complete Guide to the Healing Art*, Crossing Press, Freedom (1995).
6. Heptinstall, S. (1988) Feverfew —an ancient remedy for modern times. *J Royal Soc Med* 81:373 374.
7. Waller, P.C., Ramsay, L.E., Hylands, D.M., Johnson E.S., Kadam N.P., McRae, K.D. (1985) Efficacy of feverfew as prophylactic treatment of migraine. *Br Med J* 291: 1128.
8. Murphy, J.J., Heptinstall, S., Mitchell, I.R.A. (1988) Randomised double-blind placebo-controlled trial of feverfew in migraine prevention. *Lancet* 11: 189 192.
9. Bohimann, F., Zdero, C. (1982) Sesquiterpene lactones and other constituents from *Tanacetum parthenium*. *Phytochemistry* 21: 2643.
10. Pugh, W.J., Sambo, K. (1988) Prostaglandin synthetase inhibitors in feverfew. *J Pharm Pharmacol* 40: 743-745.

11. Collier, H.O.J., Butt, N.M., McDonald-Gibson, W.J., Saeed, S.A. (1980) Extract of feverfew inhibits prostaglandine biosynthesis. *Lancet* 11: 922-923.
12. Heptinstall, S., Williamson, L., White, A., Mitchell, J.R.H. (1985) Extracts of feverfew inhibit granule secretion in blood platelets and polymorphonuclear leucocytes. *Lancet* 1: 1071-1074.
13. Awang, D.V.C. (1987) Feverfew. Pharm J 239:487.
14. Groenewegen, W.A. (1986) Amounts of feverfew in commercial preparations of the herb. *Lancet* 1:44-45.
15. Murray, M. *Encyclopedia of Nutritional Supplements*. Prima Publishing, Rocklin, 1996.
16. Soule, Deb. *The Roots of Healing: A Woman's Book of Herbs*, Citadel Press, New York, 1995.
17. McIntyre, Anne. *The Complete Woman's Herbal*, Henry Holt Company, New York, 1994.

Resources

ASSOCIATIONS

American Association for the Study of Headaches. Referral line: 609-845-0322

American Heart Association, 7320 Greenville Avenue, Dallas, Texas 75231, (214) 373-6300.

Arthritis Foundation, 1314 Spring Street, NW, Atlanta, GA 30309, 1-800-283-7800.

National Headache Foundation, 428 W. St. James Place, Chicago, IL 60614, (800) 843-2256.

National Institute of Neurological and Communicative Disorders and Stroke, Building 31, Room 8A-06, National Institutes of Health, Bethesda, MD 20205, (301) 496-5751.

National Stroke Association, 300 East Hampden Avenue, Suite 240, Englewood, CO 80110, (303) 762-9922.

HERBAL SUPPLIERS

Seeds

Abundant Life Seed Association, P.O. Box 772, 1029 Lawrence St., Port Townsend, WA 98368.

Seeds of Change, PO Box 15700, Santa Fe, NM 87506-5700.

Herbal Products

Eclectic Institute, 11231 SE Market St., Portland, OR 97216.

Gaia Herbs, 62 Old Littleton Road, Harvard, MA 01451.

HerbPharm, 347 East Fork Road, Williams, OR 97544.

Herbalist & Alchemist Inc., P.O. Box 553, Broadway, NJ 08808, (908) 689-9020.

Herbs Etc., 1340 Rubina Circle, Santa Fe, MN 87501.

Nature's Way Products, 10 Mountain Springs Parkway, P.O. Box 2233, Springville, UT 84663.

Rainbow Light Nutritional Systems, 207 McPherson St., Santa Cruz, CA 95060.

Simpler's Botanical, P.O. Box 39, Forestville, CA 95436.

Traditional Medicinal Herb Tea Company, Sebastopol, CA 95472.

Wind River, P.O. Box 3876, Jackson, WY 83001.

Bulk Herbs

Blessed Herbs, 109 Barre Plains Road, Oakham, MA 01068.

Frontier Cooperative Herbs, Box 299, Norway, IA 52318.

Mountain Rose, P.O. Box 2000, Redway, CA 95560.

Trinity Herbs, P.O. Box 199, Bodega, CA 94992.

Pacific Botanicals, 4350 Fish Hatchery Rd., Grants Pass, OR 97527.

INDEX